Phone Numbers

School name: _____

    Phone number: _____

Mom's work phone number: _____

Dad's work phone number: _____

Other friends, family, baby sitter that might help:

Name: _____

    Phone number: _____

Name: _____

    Phone number: _____

Your child's asthma triggers: _____

_____

_____

_____

Your child's early signs of an asthma attack: _____

_____

_____

_____

_____

Dates of asthma attacks: _____

_____

_____

_____

Keep a copy of your child's Asthma Action Plan with this book.

What To Do When Your Child Has Asthma

Easy to Read • Easy to Use

Stanley P. Galant, M.D.
Olga L. Guijon, M.D.

Institute for Healthcare Advancement
501 S. Idaho St., Suite 300
La Habra, California 90631
(800) 434-4633

Institute for Healthcare Advancement
501 S. Idaho Street, Suite 300
La Habra, California 90631

Printed in the United States of America
14 13 12 11   5 4 3 2
ISBN: 978-0-9720148-6-1

To Our Readers

If your child has asthma, this book is for you. We know it's **not** easy to care for a child with asthma. There's a lot to think about every day. There are good days and bad days. We hope this book helps you keep good control of your child's asthma. Learning about asthma will help you, your child, and your family.

Each chapter in this book answers 5 questions:

- What is it?
- What do I need to know?
- What should I keep in mind?
- What can I do at home?
- When do I call the doctor or nurse?

Here are some ways to use this book:

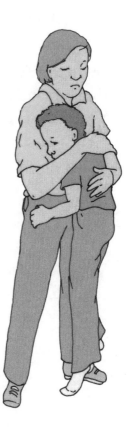

- Fill in the phone numbers in the front of the book. Keep the book where you can find it.
- Turn to page viii and read "What's in This Book."
- Read a few pages every day. Share this book with your family and others who care for your child.
- Look in the book to find answers to questions about taking care of your child.

- Take the book with you to your child's doctor visits. Ask a doctor or nurse about things in the book that you don't understand.
- When you need to give a new medicine, find the pages about that medicine. Read and learn about the medicine.
- Use the extra space in the book to write notes about your child. For example:
  - Peak flow numbers
  - The date and time your child had an asthma attack
  - Your child's asthma triggers
- Read page vii, "When to Get Help Right Away."
- See the "Word List" on page 139. You can find the meanings of many words used in the book.

The doctors who wrote this book have been treating kids with asthma for many years. Some things in this book might not be right for your child. You must decide when to call the doctor or go to an emergency room. If your child is sick and you have questions, call the doctor. Always do what your doctor or nurse says.

When to Get Help Right Away

For your child: Get help right away for any of these signs. <u>Can't</u> reach your doctor? Then call 911 or go to an emergency room.

- Child is breathing faster than normal.
- The skin is sucked in between your child's ribs or at the throat.
- Child is struggling for breath and has trouble talking. They **can't** count to 10 without taking a deep breath.
- Child coughs without stopping.
- Child's lips or nails are blue.
- The peak flow meter is in the red color zone.

For your baby: Get help right away for any of these signs. <u>Can't</u> reach your doctor? Then call 911 or go to an emergency room.

- Baby is breathing faster than normal.
- Baby stops sucking or feeding. Baby grunts during feeding due to trouble breathing.
- The skin over your baby's ribs is pulled tight.
- Baby's chest gets bigger.
- Baby's color is pale, or red in the face.
- Baby's fingertips are blue.
- Baby's cry is shorter or softer.

What's in This Book

What You Need to Know About Asthma

1

Notes

_____
_____
_____
_____
_____
_____
_____
_____
_____
_____
_____
_____
_____
_____
_____

If You Think Your Child Might Have Asthma

What is it?

Asthma (**az**-ma) is an illness of the airways in the lungs. Kids with asthma cough a lot or have trouble breathing. They make a whistling sound when they breathe.

What should I know?

The medical word for airway is bronchial (**bron**-key-ul) tube. Your doctor might say your child has "bronchial asthma." More kids have asthma today than ever before. Most doctors wait until the child is at least 2 years old before they say for sure that a child has asthma.

Asthma:

- Can happen at any age.
- Often runs in families. If a child's mom or dad has asthma, there's a greater chance the child will have it.
- Has **no** cure, but can be **controlled**.
- **Isn't** "in the child's head." Emotional problems **don't** cause asthma.
- **Isn't** something your child can "outgrow," but often can be less of a problem as the child grows.

Your child might have asthma if they:

- Have more than 2 chest colds a year.
- Have had bronchitis (bron-**kite**-iss) more than once.
- Have had pneumonia (new-**moan**-yuh) more than once.

If You Think Your Child Might Have Asthma

Asthma is a chronic (**kron**-ik) illness in most kids. That means it can come and go all your life. It **never** completely goes away. But you can control asthma with the right treatment.

If your child has asthma:

- Without good care, your child might have trouble in school. Playing sports and keeping up with other kids might be hard, too.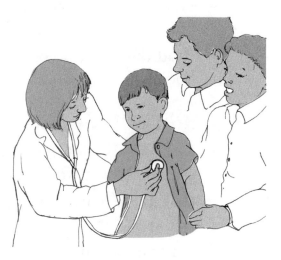

- Your doctor will tell you how to help your child once you find out he or she has asthma.

- Work with your doctor to learn how to treat and care for your child's asthma. Then your child **won't** be sick all the time.

What should I keep in mind?

- Does your child have many colds that last a long time? If so, your child might have asthma.

- A kid might **not** get over asthma as they grow older.

- **Don't** wait. Get medical help for your child. Do it as soon as you think your child has asthma.

- With a doctor's help, your child can have a normal life.

If You Think Your Child Might Have Asthma

What can I do at home?

- Plan to take your child to a doctor. Find out if your child has asthma.

- Learn how to keep your child well.

- Have a plan for taking care of your child. Your doctor can give you a written plan to follow.

- Read this book. Keep it where you can find it. This book will help you learn how to help your child.

When do I call the doctor or nurse?

- Make an appointment if you think your child has asthma. **Don't** wait until your child is sick.

- Call to ask where you can learn more about asthma.

- Call to ask if there's a local support group for parents of kids with asthma.

Asthma

What is it?

Asthma is an illness that makes it hard to breathe in or out. Your child might cough and wheeze when asthma signs start.

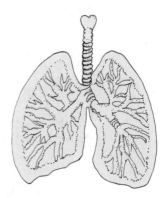

What should I know?

Asthma signs can come and go. They come more often when asthma is **not** in good control.

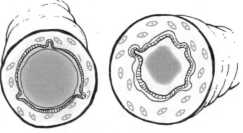

Asthma makes 3 things happen:

- The airway tubes and lungs get red and swollen (inflamed).
- Mucus (**myoo**-kus) blocks the air tubes. Mucus is a thick liquid your body makes. It protects the nose, throat, and airways. When asthma gets bad, there's too much mucus.
- Muscles around the airways get tight and squeeze the airways. This is called a "spasm."

When all this happens, air **can't** get in or out of the lungs. It feels like trying to breathe through a pinched straw.

Asthma might look like this:

- Your child has trouble getting their breath.

- They might make a whistling noise when breathing. This is called "wheezing."
- Some kids say their chest feels "tight" or "achy." They might say it feels like "someone is sitting on my chest."

Even if your child is breathing fine, their airways might be inflamed and sore. (The medical word for airway is "bronchial tube.")

Your doctor can give you medicine to help your child breathe. Asthma can be controlled.

Your doctor might use medicine or a breathing test to see if your child has asthma.

A bronchodilator (bronk-oh-**die**-late-er) is a medicine that makes the airways relax and open up. Your child might have asthma if they get better right after using a bronchodilator.

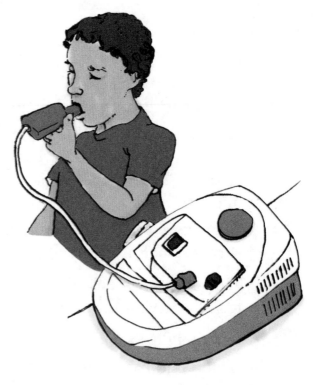

When a child is age 5 or more, your doctor might use a spirometer (spi-**rom**-e-ter) to check for asthma. The spirometer will check the amount of air going in and out of the lungs. This test does **not** hurt.

What should I keep in mind?

- Trouble breathing is caused by red and swollen airways.
- The airways are blocked by mucus.
- The muscles are tight around the airways.
- Medicine will make the child feel better. It will make the airways less tight so your child can breathe.
- If your child is 5 years or older, your doctor might use a spirometer to see if they have asthma.

What can I do at home?

- Learn about asthma.
- Learn what your child's early asthma signs are so you can give medicine before the asthma gets worse.
- Read this book to learn how to care for your child.
- Talk to your family about your child's asthma. Teach other adults who care for your child about asthma.
- Plan to take your child to the doctor. The doctor will tell you what to do for your child.

When do I call the doctor or nurse?

- Make an appointment to see the doctor if you think your child's asthma signs are coming too often. (To learn about the Rules of 2, see page 11.)
- Call whenever you need to know more about asthma.

Asthma Signs

What is it?

Asthma signs are things you might fell, see, or hear when your child has asthma. Signs (such as wheezing) are **not** always visible.

What should I know?

The main signs of asthma are:

- Wheezing. This is a whistling sound in the chest when breathing out. Sometimes you can hear it when your child breathes in.
- Trouble breathing or trouble getting a full breath.
- A cough that **doesn't** go away, like these:
  - Dry hacking cough
  - Cough that's **not** just from a cold or flu
  - Cough in the middle of the night
  - Cough after playing hard, running around, or playing sports

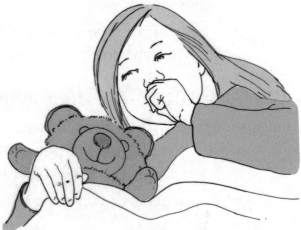

Your child might have asthma even if they **don't** have the main signs of asthma.

Here are some other signs that your child might have asthma:

- Child's chest feels tight like a drum.
- Breathing is fast.
- Child has to work hard to breathe.
- Child is tired a lot.
- Child has trouble sleeping.

Kids under 5 years old **can't** always tell you what's wrong. You'll have to watch a younger child more closely.

Signs that young children are having trouble with their asthma are:

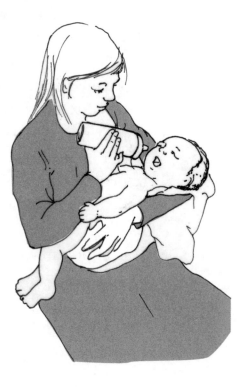

- Breathing is fast.
- The nostrils on the child's nose are open wide.
- Child is **not** eating or has trouble eating. Child **can't** suck.
- The skin is sucked in between the child's ribs.
- Child's cry is soft and short.
- There is no color in the child's face.
- Child's fingertips are blue.

If your child has any of these signs, see a doctor right away.

What should I keep in mind?

- Wheezing might be a sign that your child has asthma.
- Your child might have asthma if they always have a cough.
- A cough that often happens in the middle of the night might be a sign that your child has asthma.
- A cough when playing hard might be a sign that your child has asthma.
- Some kids have allergies that can make asthma signs start. **Not** all kids with allergies have asthma. Your doctor will tell you.
- Children with asthma should have bronchodilator medicine to help them feel better when signs start. This is called rescue (**RES**-kyue) or quick-relief medicine.
- Some children might need a controller medicine to better control their asthma symptoms. Your doctor can tell you if your child needs a controller medicine. (See "Controller Medicine – Inhaled Corticosteroids," page 57.)
- It is important to learn about your child's medicines.
- Only your doctor can tell you if your child has asthma.

What can I do at home?

- Learn about your child's asthma signs.
- Learn what brings on your child's asthma signs.
- Know how and when to give your child their asthma medicine.
- Ask your doctor for a written plan that tells how to help your child.

- Learn the "Rules of 2." Your child's asthma is **not** under control if:
  - Asthma signs come 2 or more days a week.
  - Asthma signs that come at night more than 1 or 2 times a month.
  - Your child needs to have their quick-relief medicine refilled more than 2 times a year.

When do I call the doctor or nurse?

- Call if you think your child has asthma.
- Call when you **don't** know how to care for your child.
- When your child has the signs of asthma, follow the asthma plan. Call your child's doctor right away. Give your child quick-relief medicine. If it does **not** help, call 911 or go to an emergency room.

Asthma Attack

What is it?

An asthma attack is when your child's early signs of asthma get worse.

What should I know?

An asthma attack can happen all at once, with no warning.

Sometimes there are warning signs. Your child might:
- Get a cold in the chest.
- Cough more at night.
- Wheeze more at night.
- Play less or stop playing at all.
- Have an itchy or scratchy throat.
- Have a stuffy or runny nose.
- Act more tired than usual.
- Breathe faster than normal.

Learn how fast your child breathes **before** they have an asthma attack. Then you'll know when your child is breathing faster than normal.

There are 5 ways to tell if your child is having a bad attack. If your child has any of these, **give the quick-relief medicine. Then call 911, or go to an emergency room. Get medical help right away.**

1. Is your child breathing faster than normal? Too fast is:

   - **Babies under 2 years old**— more than 40 times a minute at rest.
   - **Kids 2 to 10 years old**—more than 30 times a minute at rest.
   - **Kids older than 10**—more than 20 times a minute at rest.

If you're **not** sure how many breaths your child is taking, call your doctor or 911.

2. Is the skin sucking in between the ribs or at the front of your child's neck?

3. Is your child short of breath? Are they having trouble talking?

4. Does your child cough without stopping?

5. Are your child's lips and fingertips blue?

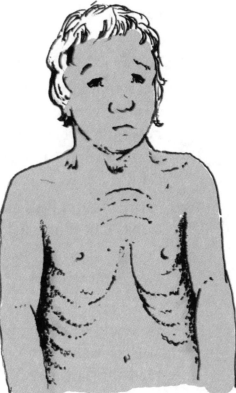

Not all kids have the same signs of asthma.

Your doctor will help you get good control of your child's asthma. With good control, asthma attacks **don't** happen often.

What should I keep in mind?

- **A bad attack is an emergency. Call your doctor right away. If you <u>can't</u> reach the doctor right away, call 911 or take your child to an emergency room. <u>Don't</u> wait.**
- Know the early signs of an asthma attack.
- Use this book to check the list of early signs of an asthma attack.
- When you see signs of asthma, give your child the medicine your doctor told you to give.
- Work with your child's doctor to control asthma.
- Work with the doctor to stop asthma attacks when they happen.

What can I do at home?

- Learn when your child is having an asthma attack. Make a list of your child's early signs so you can help before it gets worse. Tape the list where you can see it easily. Try putting it on the inside of a kitchen cupboard door or on the fridge.
- Write your child's asthma signs on the first page of this book. Check the list when you think your child might be having an asthma attack.
- Notice how your child breathes when they are well. Then you'll know what's normal.
- Be ready to take care of your child during an asthma attack. Make sure you always have your child's medicines ready and nearby.

- Give your child the medicines your doctor has told you to give for quick relief.

- Learn the "Rules of 2." Your child's asthma is **not** under control if:

  - Asthma signs come 2 or more days a week.

  - Asthma signs that come at night more than 1 or 2 times a month.

  - Your child needs to have their quick-relief medicine refilled more than 2 times a year.

- Is your child's peak flow less than 2 times 10 (20%) from baseline or in the yellow zone of their Asthma Action Plan with asthma symptoms?

If you can answer "Yes" to any of these questions, your child's asthma is **not** under control.

- Write down phone numbers to call for help when your child is having an asthma attack. Put the numbers in the front of this book.

When do I call the doctor or nurse?

- Call your doctor when you're **not** sure if your child is having an asthma attack. If you **can't** reach your doctor right away, call 911 or go to an emergency room.

- Call if you're **not** sure how to care for your child during an asthma attack.

- Call anytime you feel your child is **not** OK and needs medical help.

- When your child is having a bad asthma attack, call 911 or go to the emergency room.

Taking Charge of Your Child's Asthma

2

Notes

_____

_____

_____

_____

_____

_____

_____

_____

_____

_____

_____

_____

_____

_____

Asthma Triggers

What is it?

A trigger is something that brings on asthma signs in your child.

What should I know?

Triggers are things that make the airways in your child's lungs red and swollen. This is called "inflammation" (in-flah-**may**-shun). **Not** every child with asthma has the same triggers.

Staying away from triggers will help your child's asthma. Your child should need less quick-relief medicine if they stay away from their triggers.

- **Cold air** can trigger asthma.
- **Flu or a cold** might trigger asthma.
- **Exercise** can also trigger asthma.
- **Allergens** (**al**-ler-jens) and other things in the air can trigger asthma.

An allergen is something that bothers some people, but not all. Allergens can cause inflammation in your child's body. See below for a list of allergens.

When your child breathes in or eats an allergen, they might get signs of allergy.

Here are some signs of allergy:

- Runny nose

- Rash
- Coughing or sneezing
- Wheezing
- Itchy nose, eyes, or skin
- Trouble breathing
- Swollen lips or eyelids

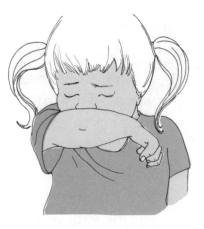

Allergic triggers can make your child cranky, unhappy, or restless.

There are **indoor** allergens and **outdoor** allergens.

Allergens **inside** your home that can trigger asthma are:

- **Dust mites.** Dust mites are smaller than the tip of a pin. You **can't** see dust mites. Dust mites live in carpets, mattresses, pillows, and bedding. Dust mites are in the air, too. Many children with asthma are allergic to dust mites even if they **don't** have other allergies.

- **Pet dander.** Pet dander is **not** hair. Pet dander is small, dead skin cells shed by animals. The dander floats in the air. Dander lands on furniture. Dander becomes a part of dust. You **can't** see dander. Pet drool and pee also trigger asthma. There is no such thing as a dog or cat that does **not** have dander.

- **Mold.** Mold is a fungus. Molds like damp and wet places best, but they are everywhere. Molds are in the air. Molds are easy to breathe in. They are in your home and outdoors. They are in your child's school.

- **Cockroaches.** The bowel movements (BM) and spit of cockroaches are in house dust.

19

Allergens in the air **outside** your home that can trigger asthma are:

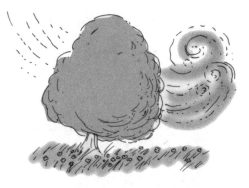

- **Pollen** from trees and weeds. This trigger happens in the spring and fall months.

- **Pollen** from grass. This happens mostly in the summer months.

- **Molds** in dirt, grass, fall leaves, and air. They cause symptoms mainly in the fall months.

Food might be an allergen. Food allergens are sometimes more dangerous than air allergens.

Here are some food allergens:

- Peanuts and other nuts
- Cow's milk
- Egg white
- Soy
- Wheat
- Fish and shellfish
- Sesame seeds

Other things in the air can trigger asthma. These are called "irritants."

Here are some irritants in the air that might trigger asthma:

- Smoke from cigarettes, cigars, incense, or pipes
- Fireplace smoke

- Smog
- Fumes from a factory
- Strong smells
- Sprays used on hair or for cleaning and air fresheners

What should I keep in mind?

- Look for things that trigger your child's asthma. If you know a trigger, you can work at getting rid of it.
- Get rid of triggers to help your child stay well.

What can I do at home?

- Ask yourself and your family these questions. Write the answers down. Show them to your doctor:
  - Does your child's asthma get worse during the week when your child is at school?
  - Does your child's asthma get worse during cold or wet weather?
  - Does your child's asthma get worse at the same time each year?
  - Does your child's asthma get worse after playing with a cat or dog?
  - Does your child's asthma get worse after eating some kinds of food?
  - Does your child's asthma get worse when they play or exercise?
- Vacuum and dust your home every day if you can.

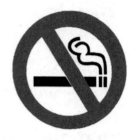

- Remove carpets if you can. It is best if your child's bedroom does **not** have one.

- **Don't** let people smoke in your home, in your car, or around your child.

- Try **not** to have pets in your home, at least **not** in your child's bedroom.

- Wash your hands often. Teach your child to wash **their** hands often, too.

- Get rid of dust mites:

  - Use dustproof covers with zippers on your child's pillows and mattress.

  - Remove the bedroom carpet. If you **can't** remove it, vacuum it every day. Vacuum the furniture once a week.

  - Wash bedding in hot water once a week. Dry the bedding completely.

  - Buy only stuffed toys that you can wash. Let them dry before your child plays with them again. Try **not** to keep more than 3 in your child's bedroom.

- Get rid of mold:

  - Remove carpets that are always damp or wet. A hard floor and a throw rug are best.

  - Repair water leaks as soon as you can.

  - Clean mold from hard surfaces with soap and water. Let them dry.

  - **Don't** use a vaporizer or humidifier in your child's bedroom. These are hard to clean well.

- Get rid of cockroaches. Use roach baits or traps. **Don't** leave food or spills on the counter or floors. Take the trash out of the home to the trash can. Keep a lid on the trash can.
- **Don't** let your child share cups, spoons, or towels with other kids.
- Wash your child's toys. Use soap and water.
- **Don't** use scented candles, incense, air fresheners, or scented room sprays.
- Avoid giving your child foods that trigger their asthma.
- Make sure your child takes the medicine the doctor orders.

When do I call the doctor or nurse?

- Call when you **don't** know what to do about your child's asthma triggers.

Asthma Severity Levels

What is it?

Asthma severity (seh-**ver**-i-tee) describes different levels of asthma. Your child's level tells you how bad your child's asthma is. Knowing the level helps the doctor decide the next step to help your child. Your doctor decides the severity levels when your child first gets asthma.

What should I know?

Know how often your child has asthma signs. Know how long the signs last. Tell your child's doctor. This will help your doctor start a treatment plan for your child.

Your doctor will ask questions to decide if your child has **intermittent** asthma or **persistent** asthma.

- **Intermittent** (in-ter-**mitt**-ent) is when your child has asthma **only once in awhile**.
- **Persistent** (per-**sis**-tent) is when your child has asthma symptoms more often.

Intermittent asthma and **persistent** asthma are **not** treated the same way. Kids with **intermittent** asthma **don't** need daily medicine to control asthma. They only need a quick-relief medicine less than 2 days a week.

Kids with **persistent** asthma **do** need to take controller medicine every day. It is important to remember that even if they **don't** have signs of asthma very often, they need their medicine every day. Having less asthma signs is the goal! It means the controller medicine is working.

Asthma Severity Levels

Your doctor will ask these questions at every visit to check how well the medicine is working. Be ready to answer as many as you can:

- How many days a week does your child have signs of asthma?
- How many times each month do they wake up at night with asthma?
- Does asthma make your child stop playing or exercising?
- How many times did your child need quick-relief medicine for asthma?
- What are your child's peak flow numbers (if your child has a peak flow meter)? (See "Peak Flow Meter and the Asthma Action Plan," page 32.)

What should I keep in mind?

- There are different levels of asthma, called Asthma Severity Levels.
- Each level is treated differently.
- Your doctor will know your child's level of asthma and treat it.
- Your doctor will tell you what medicines to give your child.

What can I do at home?

- Get rid of asthma triggers from your home.
- Notice how often your child has signs of asthma. Write down answers to these questions. Tell your child's doctor:
  - Do the signs of asthma happen in the daytime or at night?

- How often does your child have trouble breathing?
- How often does your child need quick-relief medicine?

- Tell everyone at home about your child's asthma, and what to do for it. Tell teachers, school nurses, babysitters, and other family members, too.

- Know your doctor's plan for when your child should take medicine. Make a list. Put the list where everyone can see it.

- Show everyone in your family how to call 911.

When do I call the doctor or nurse?

- Call when what you are doing for your child **doesn't** help.

- Call if your child's asthma gets worse.

- Call if you **can't** give your child the medicine the doctor told you to give.

- Call if you **don't** have the medicine you need.

- Should you call if your child is having a bad asthma attack? Yes. Give quick-relief medicine. Then **call 911** or go to the emergency room.

Asthma Control

What is it?

Controlling asthma is doing things that help prevent asthma symptoms and asthma attacks. Good control, means few or no asthma symptoms or attacks.

What should I know?

Good control of asthma will prevent more problems for your child. It will help your child have normal lung growth.

Good control is what every doctor tries to do.

Learn the "Rules of 2." Your child's asthma is **not** under control if:

- Asthma signs come 2 or more days a week.
- Asthma signs that come at night more than 1 or 2 times a month.
- Your child needs to have their quick-relief medicine refilled more than 2 times a year.

When your child has good asthma control, your child will:

- Sleep through the night without waking up.
- Keep up with other children.
- Play **without** having trouble breathing.
- **Not** miss school. (**You** won't miss work.)
- Have **no** emergency room visits for asthma.

You need to work closely with your child's doctor to have good asthma control.

What should I keep in mind?

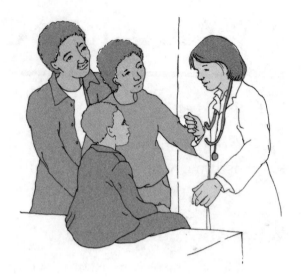

- You can control your child's asthma.

- You need to work with the doctor on a plan for your child.

- When asthma is controlled, your child will have a normal life.

- If the doctor gives your child controller medicines, your child must use them **every day**. Their airways are still inflamed, even when you **don't** see signs of asthma.

What can I do at home?

- Keep asthma triggers out of your home.
- Follow the plan for caring for your child's asthma.
- Give your child the medicine the doctor has prescribed.
- Talk to everyone in your family about how to control your child's asthma.
- Teach your child about asthma. Help your child learn how to control their asthma.

When do I call the doctor or nurse?

- Call when you **can't** do what the asthma plan tells you to.
- Call if you think your child has a problem with allergies.
- Call if your child's asthma gets worse.
- Call to learn what to do when your child goes to school.
- Call if you have any questions about your child's medicine.
- Call if your family wants you to give medicine that your doctor **didn't** tell you to use.

Planning to Care for Your Child's Asthma

3

Notes

_____

_____

_____

_____

_____

_____

_____

_____

_____

_____

_____

_____

_____

_____

Peak Flow Meter and the Asthma Action Plan

What is it?

A peak flow meter is a tool. It tells how well your child is breathing.

What should I know?

A peak flow meter tells how much air your child breathes out at one time. You can use it with kids 5 years old or older. The child holds the peak flow meter in their hand.

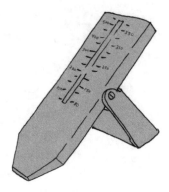

Many kids **can't** tell when they're having trouble breathing. A peak flow meter can let you know that your child is having trouble. You can then give medicine right away. You might **not** need to go to an emergency room.

Your child blows into the meter 3 times. You write down each number the pointer goes to. This number tells how much air your child breathed out.

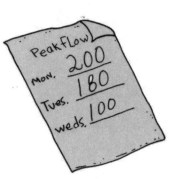

The highest number you write down is the number you'll use on your child's Asthma Action Plan. (See "Asthma Action Plan," page 42.)

Peak Flow Meter and the Asthma Action Plan

How to use a peak flow meter

Have pen and paper ready. Tell your child to stand or sit up straight.

1. For practice, have your child breathe with their mouth open. Tell them to breathe in and out. Have them breathe as much air as they can 2 times.

2. Move the pointer on the peak flow meter to 0.

3. Put the mouthpiece flat on your child's tongue. Have your child close their lips tightly around the mouthpiece.

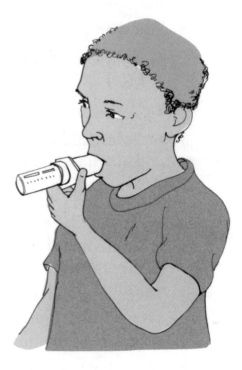

4. Tell your child to take a deep breath. Your child then blows out as fast and hard as they can.

5. Find the number where the pointer stops.

6. Move the pointer back to 0.

7. Wait 15 seconds.

8. Do this 2 more times.

9. Write down the highest of the 3 numbers. This is your child's best score.

What should I keep in mind?

- The peak flow number can tell you if your child's airway is closing down. It can let you know when to give your child more medicine.

- Ask your doctor to give you a written **Asthma Action Plan** that shows how to take care of your child's asthma. If your child uses a peak flow meter, ask your doctor to include the peak flow numbers for your child on the plan. Learn what to do when your child has a number that is low.

- You **won't** get a correct reading if:
  - Your child has gum in their mouth.
  - Your child spits or coughs when they blow.
  - Your child puts their tongue over the mouthpiece.
  - Your child forces air out for too long.
  - Your child blows too slowly or **doesn't** try their best.
  - Your child's fingers cover the vent or stop the pointer from moving.
  - Your child **doesn't** keep their lips tight around the mouthpiece.

- There are different kinds of peak flow meters. Ask your doctor which kind you should use. A "low-range" meter is better for a young child.

- You can get a peak flow meter at the doctor's office, a clinic, or the drugstore. Make sure they show your child how to use the meter. Practice with your child to make sure your child is using it the right way.

- Have your child use the meter while the doctor watches. Ask the doctor if your child did it right. Make sure your child is using the meter the right way before you leave the doctor's office.
- You **don't** need a prescription to buy a peak flow meter. But ask a pharmacist to help you pick which one to buy. Have them show you how to use it.

What can I do at home?

- Try to use the peak flow meter at the same time every day.
- Also use the peak flow meter when you think your child is having asthma signs.
- You should watch your child use a peak flow meter until they are 14 years old. Make sure your child is using the peak flow meter the right way. Make sure your child uses the meter for 3 times to get the highest number.
- Teach family members how to use the peak flow meter.
- Write down your child's peak flow numbers. Note the **best** of the 3 numbers. Take your child's peak flow numbers with you when you go to the doctor.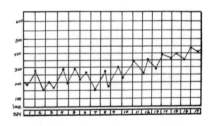
- Keep the peak flow meter clean. Once a week, wash the outside with warm water and let it air dry. **Don't** use soap or brushes to wash it. Do **not** touch the inside of your peak flow meter.
- Keep your child's peak flow meter in a zip lock plastic bag.

Peak Flow Meter and the Asthma Action Plan

- Keep the peak flow meter in the same place every time. That way, you'll know where it is when you need it.

- You might want 2 peak flow meters: 1 for home and 1 for school. When you use 2 meters, buy the same brand.

When do I call the doctor or nurse?

- Call if you **don't** know how to use a peak flow meter.

- **Call if your child <u>can't</u> move the pointer on the peak flow meter above half of their best number. If you <u>can't</u> reach the doctor right away, call 911 or go to the emergency room. <u>Don't</u> wait.**

Personal Best Peak Flow Number

What is it?

The personal best peak flow number is the highest number your child reaches using a peak flow meter for **2 weeks**. It tells how much air your child breathes in and out on their best day.

What should I know?

- You need to find your child's personal best peak flow number. To do this, use a peak flow meter when your child is **not** having signs of asthma.

- Take the peak flow measure 2 times a day. Do it once in the morning and once in the evening. Write down the peak flow numbers. (See "Peak Flow Meter and the Asthma Action Plan," page 32.)

- Do this for 2 weeks. The highest number over 2 weeks is your child's personal best.

- The personal best peak flow number is important. This is the **best** number your child gets on the meter. Tell your doctor this number.

- Your child's personal best helps your doctor know what asthma medicine to give your child and **when**.

- The personal best peak flow number will get bigger as your child grows.

- Get your child's personal best peak flow number every 12 months. Measure more often if:
  - Your child has a growth spurt OR
  - Their asthma gets worse.

What can I do at home?

For the 2-week period

- Learn how your child should use a peak flow meter.
- Plan a time in the morning and evening to use the peak flow meter.
- Use the meter at the same times every day for 2 weeks.
- Keep a peak flow book. Write down the day of the week, the time of day, and the peak flow number.

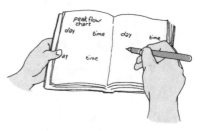

After the 2-week period

- After your child's Asthma Action Plan has been written with these numbers, you only need to check Peak Flow when your child shows signs of asthma.

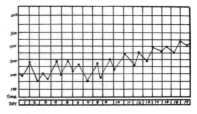

When do I call the doctor or nurse?

- Call if you **can't** get your child to use the peak flow meter.
- Call for an appointment to talk about your child's personal best peak flow meter number.

Peak Flow Meter Color Zone System

What is it?

The written asthma plan has a Color Zone System. It uses traffic light colors. The color zones tell you what to do for your child's asthma. The asthma plan can be used even if your child **doesn't** have a peak flow meter.

What should I know?

Your doctor will use a Color Zone System to tell you what to do for your child.

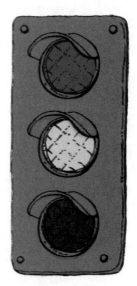

- The **green color zone** means your child's asthma is in good control. Your child does **not** have signs of asthma. Keep giving prescribed controller medicines.

- The **yellow color zone** means you should watch your child closely. Your child's asthma might **not** be under control. The doctor might need to change or add to your child's medicines.

- The **red color zone** means danger. Your child needs to see a doctor right away.

Your doctor will write your child's numbers for each color zone. The numbers go under "Peak Flow Percent of Personal Best." Match your child's peak flow meter number to the number the doctor has written. See which color zone your child is in.

Peak Flow Meter Color Zone System

Your doctor will tell you what to do when your child is in the green, yellow, or red color zone. This will help you when the peak flow number changes.

Peak Flow Color Zone System
(Ask your doctor to fill in your child's numbers.)

Zone	What This Means	Peak Flow Percent of Personal Best
Green	Asthma in good control	80% to 100% (doctor writes here) _____
Yellow	Mild to moderate asthma attack or asthma is worse	50% to 80% (doctor writes here) _____
Red	Severe attack	Less than 50% (doctor writes here) _____

Using the 3 color zones, your doctor might tell you:

- When your child's peak flow number is in the **green zone or your child has no asthma symptoms**, use the same treatment plan.

- When the peak flow is in the **yellow zone**, give quick-relief medicine. Wait 10 minutes. Check the peak flow again. If the peak flow number **doesn't** go to the green zone, call your doctor.

- If your child's peak flow is often in the **yellow zone or your child has asthma symptoms**, call your doctor.

- If the peak flow is in the **red zone or your child has severe asthma symptoms**, give quick-relief medicine. **Call 911 or go to the emergency room.**

When do I call the doctor or nurse?

- Call if you **can't** get your child's peak flow number.
- Call if your child's peak flow is in the yellow zone after giving medicine.
- Call if your child is often in the yellow color zone.
- **When your child is in the red color zone, give quick-relief medicine. Then call 911 or go to the emergency room.**

Asthma Action Plan

What is it?

The Asthma Action Plan tells you what to do for your child's asthma.

What should I know?

Your child's doctor writes the Asthma Action Plan. If the doctor **doesn't** give you a plan, ask for one.

For kids under age 5 years:

The doctor uses your child's asthma signs to write the Asthma Action Plan.

For kids 5 years old or older:

- Personal best peak flow meter numbers (if using)
- Your child's asthma signs

The Asthma Action Plan will tell:

- Early signs of an asthma problem.
- Peak flow meter numbers for each color zone (green, yellow, and red).
- Controller medicines and how to use them.
- Quick-relief medicines and how to use them.

The plan will also tell you the steps to take for an asthma attack. It will say when to call your doctor and when to get emergency help. It will have phone numbers to use in an emergency.

The Asthma Action Plan uses 3 color zones. Your child's peak flow number will fall into one of these color zones. (See "Peak Flow Meter Color Zone System," page 39.)

- **Green color zone means:**
  - Peak flow at 80-100% of personal best flow. Your doctor will tell you the number for the green zone. Ask your doctor to write it in the chart on page 45.
  - No asthma signs.
  - Daily controller medicine and how much to give your child.

- **Yellow color zone means:**
  - Peak flow at 50-80% of personal best flow. Your doctor will tell you the number for the yellow zone. Ask your doctor to write it in the chart on page 45.
  - Signs include coughing, wheezing, tight chest, or waking up at night with a cough.
  - Child is in the yellow zone when they need quick-relief medicine more than 2 times a week. **Your child should <u>not</u> use quick-relief medicine every day.**
  - Give your child quick-relief medicine and continue controller medicine.
  - **Call the doctor if asthma signs <u>don't</u> get better and stay better for more than 1 day.**

- **Red color zone means:**
  - Peak flow is less than 50%. Your doctor will tell you the number for the red zone. Ask the doctor to write it in the chart on page 45.

- Child has signs of asthma:
  - Child is breathing faster than normal.
  - The skin is sucked in between your child's ribs or at the throat.
  - Child is struggling for breath and has trouble talking.
  - Child coughs without stopping.
  - Child's lips or nails are blue.
- Quick-relief medicine **doesn't** help.
- **Go to an emergency room or call 911. <u>Don't</u> wait.**

Using an Asthma Action Plan

- Find which color zone your child is in:
  - What is your child's peak flow number?
  - Does your child have signs of asthma?
- Look across from your child's color zone to know what to do for your child.

Here is what an Asthma Action Plan might look like. Your doctor might use an Asthma Action Plan that is **not** the same. Most plans use color zones and tell you what to do for your child.

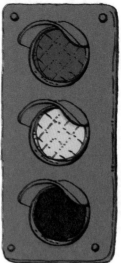

Asthma Action Plan

Asthma Action Plan			
GREEN ZONE **GO** Peak flow is from: _____ to _____ • Breathing is OK • No cough or wheeze • Can run and play • Sleeps through the night	**Take these medicines every day**		
	Medicine	How Much	How Often
	Before exercise _____		
YELLOW ZONE **CAUTION** Peak flow is from: _____ to _____ If you have any of these: • Cough • Wheeze • Tight chest • Waking up at night with a cough	**Add these and keep taking the green zone medicine**		
	Medicine	How Much	How Often
RED ZONE **DANGER** Peak flow is below ____ • Medicine is not helping • Breathes fast and hard • Ribs show • Can't walk • Can't talk well • Coughs all the time • Lips or nails are blue	**Take these medicines and call your doctor now or call 911!**		
	Medicine	How Much	How Often

What should I keep in mind?

Your child's Asthma Action Plan will:

- Tell you the best way to treat your child's asthma.
- Tell you what to do when your child's asthma gets worse.
- Help you take charge of your child's asthma.

What can I do at home?

- Make sure you understand the Asthma Action Plan for your child.
- Make sure everyone who cares for your child understands the plan. **This includes babysitters.**
- Make copies of your child's Asthma Action Plan.
- Put a copy of the plan:
  - Near your child's bed.
  - Where you keep your child's medicines.
  - On the fridge door.
  - Near your phone.
  - In your car.
- Take a copy of the Asthma Action Plan with you when you travel.
- Bring the Asthma Action Plan to the doctor or ER.
- Make sure teachers, school nurse, coaches, and other group leaders have a copy of the plan.

- Learn your child's early asthma signs. Look for things like:
  - Changes in breathing.
  - Coughing at night.
  - **Not** wanting to play.
  - Coughing when playing or laughing.
  - Saying their chest hurts or feels funny.
  - Scratchy or itchy throat.
  - Waking up at night with wheezing.
- Help your child learn all about their Asthma Action Plan. Make sure your child is following their Asthma Action Plan. As your child grows, teach them to care for their asthma on their own.
- Keep your child's asthma triggers out of your home and other places your child visits.
- Have a routine for using the peak flow meter and giving medicine. Do this so you **won't** forget to give your child medicine. Do this even when your child is feeling well. Do it so your child understands this is what **they** need to do.

When do I call the doctor or nurse?

- Call anytime you **don't** know what to do for your child.
- Call anytime you **can't** give your child their medicine.
- Call if your child is often in the yellow zone.
- **When your child is in the red zone, give them quick-relief medicine. Then call 911 or go to the emergency room right away.**

Your Child's Asstma Medicines

4

Notes

_____

_____

_____

_____

_____

_____

_____

_____

_____

_____

_____

_____

_____

Asthma Medicine

What is it?

Asthma medicines control and treat asthma.

What should I know?

There are 3 types of asthma medicine:

- Controller
- Quick-relief
- Oral steroids (**ster**-oidz)

Your child's Asthma Action Plan will tell you when to use each medicine.

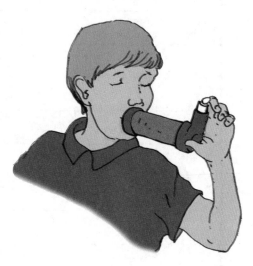

- **Controller medicine:**
  - Use it every day. Inhaled controller medicines are usually given twice a day.
  - Give it even when there are **no** signs of asthma.
  - This medicine makes your child's airways less swollen.
  - It helps prevent an asthma attack.
  - It might take several weeks to start working.
  - Other names for this medicine are "anti-inflammatory," "long-term," or "preventive."

- See "Controller Medicine – Inhaled Corticosteroids," page 57, and "Other Controller Medicines," page 62.
- **Quick-relief medicine:**
  - Use it when your child has asthma signs.
  - Your doctor might have your child use it before exercise or gym class.
  - This medicine relaxes the muscles around the airway.
  - Your child inhales, or breathes in, this medicine. It is best to give it with a holding chamber. Holding chambers help inhaled medicine to work much better.
  - This medicine works very fast. It should help your child within minutes.
  - Another name for this medicine is "rescue" medicine.
  - See "Quick-Relief Medicine," page 54.
- **Oral steroids:**
  - Oral steroids come as a pill or syrup.
  - They reduce redness and swelling in your child's lungs.
  - Use them for a few days with bad asthma attacks.
  - Your child might need oral steroids for a longer time when other medicine **isn't** helping.
  - These medicines can cause bad side effects if you use them for weeks or months.
  - The doctor needs to see your child often when your child needs oral steroids. This way the doctor can check on side effects. They also will make sure the oral steroids work.
  - **Not** needing oral steroids is an important goal of treatment. There are far less side effects with inhaled

controller medicines. The right inhaled medicine, given as the doctor orders, should help keep your child off oral steroids.

- See "Oral Steroids," page 67.

Your doctor will tell you what medicine to use. The doctor decides based on your child's asthma symptoms and asthma severity.

Remember, your doctor will decide if your child has intermittent or persistent asthma. (See "Asthma Severity Levels," page 24.)

- For intermittent asthma, your child needs only quick-relief medicine.

- For persistent asthma, your child will need controller medicine. You'll use quick-relief medicine when needed.

What should I keep in mind?

- An Asthma Action Plan tells you how to get good control of your child's asthma.

- Work with your doctor. It's important for the doctor to know how well your child's asthma medications are working.

- Following an Asthma Action Plan can help stop asthma attacks.

- With good control, your child will have fewer asthma attacks.

- With good control, your child can do all the things other kids do.

What can I do at home?

- Keep all your child's medicines in one place. Keep them out of your child's reach.
- Always keep enough medicine on hand.
- Know each medicine your child is taking:
  - Name of the medicine
  - What the medicine is for
  - How the medicine works
  - When to give the medicine
  - Side effects of the medicine
  - How long to take the medicine
- Give daily medicines **at the same time** every day. Waiting too long might bring on signs of asthma.
- Keep everything you use to give your child medicine in one place.
- Make sure your child knows how to use their inhaler the right way.
- Keep all doctor appointments.

When do I call the doctor or nurse?

- Call the doctor if you **don't** understand your child's Asthma Action Plan.
- Call if your child **won't** take their medicine.
- Call when you need to refill your child's medicine.
- Call if the medicine **doesn't** seem to be helping your child.

Quick-Relief Medicine

What is it?

Quick-relief medicine works in minutes. It relaxes the muscles around the airway. This makes breathing easier. Quick-relief medicine usually helps with asthma signs and asthma attacks.

What should I know?

Quick-relief medicine is also called "rescue" medicine. Your child uses it when they have trouble breathing.

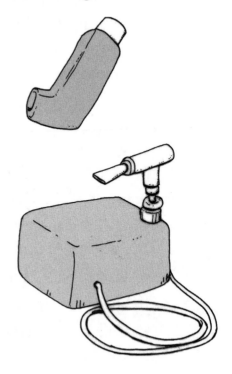

- Give quick-relief medicine when your child needs it (cough, wheeze, trouble breathing).
- Your child should feel better in 5 to 10 minutes after taking the medicine.
- Your child inhales quick-relief medicine. This means they breathe it into the lungs. It works faster than a pill or syrup.
- The doctor might want your child to take quick-relief medicine 5-15 minutes before exercise. It helps stop asthma signs for 2-4 hours.

- Quick-relief medicine **doesn't** treat inflamed lungs.
- Quick-relief medicine needs a doctor's order. You can get it as a metered-dose inhaler or a liquid. You use a holding chamber with the metered-dose inhaler. You use the liquid with a breathing machine called a "nebulizer" (neb-yoo-lye-zer).

Here are the brands and generic names of some quick-relief medicines:

- ProAir® HFA (albuterol)
- Proventil® HFA (albuterol)
- Ventolin® HFA (albuterol)
- Xopenex® HFA (levalbuterol)
- ProAir® Repiclick HFA (albuterol)

Here are some possible side effects of quick-relief medicine:

- Feeling jittery
- Shaking
- Scratchy throat
- Fast heart rate

What should I keep in mind?

- Albuterol is the right medicine when your child is having an asthma attack.
- Albuterol will start to work in 5 to 10 minutes.
- Albuterol will work in the body for up to 4 hours.
- All brands of albuterol work about the same way.
- What if your child gets shaky or has a fast heart rate after taking albuterol? The doctor might prescribe Xopenex® HFA (levalbuterol).

What should I do at home?

- Make sure you have enough quick-relief medicine for home and school. Never let it run out completely.
- Keep the quick-relief medicine where it's easy to find.
- Follow your child's Asthma Action Plan.
- **Never** give more medicine than your doctor has told you to give.

When do I call the doctor or nurse?

- Call to talk about medicine side effects your child is having.
- Call for a refill of the quick-relief medicine.
- Call your child's doctor if the medicine **isn't** helping.
- Call to ask how to take quick-relief medicine the right way.

Controller Medicine – Inhaled Corticosteroids

What is it?

Inhaled corticosteroids are medicines you breathe in. They reduce redness and swelling in the airways and lungs. They are usually the first choice of controller medicine.

What should I know?

An inhaled corticosteroid (kor-ti-ko-**ster**-oid) is a controller medicine. It might be called ICS for short. Other words used for controller medicine are "anti-inflammatory," "long term," and "preventive."

ICSs are used for persistent asthma.

- When your child uses an ICS daily:
    - Airways will **not** swell as much.
    - There will be less mucus in your child's airways.
- ICS can take up to 4-6 weeks to work fully.
- You never use ICSs for quick-relief.
- You use ICSs every day to keep your child free from asthma signs.
- Inhaled medicine goes right to the lungs. Your child will have fewer side effects with an ICS than with a pill or syrup.
- ICSs will help your child's lungs grow normally.

Controller Medicine – Inhaled Corticosteroids

Inhaled corticosteroids are given:

- With a metered-dose inhaler (MDI).
- As a dry powder inhaler.
- With a nebulizer machine.

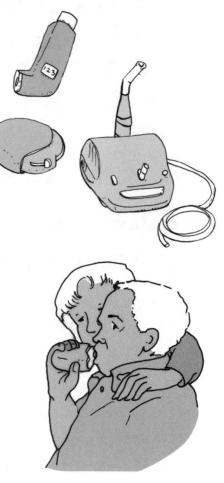

Always use a holding chamber with a metered-dose inhaler. A holding chamber is a plastic tube you put on an inhaler. It helps your child get the full dose of the medicine. You need to clean the holding chamber once a week. (Read "Using a Holding Chamber," page 82.)

Here are some inhaled corticosteroids:

- QVAR® (beclomethasone)
- Pulmicort® (budesonide)
- Alvesco® (ciclesonide)
- Flovent® HFA (fluticasone)
- Asmanex® (mometasone)
- Aerospan® (flunisolide)
- Arnuity® Ellipta (fluticasone furoate)
- Aerobid® (flunisolide)

Side effects of ICSs **aren't** common, but might include:

- Hoarse voice.
- Thrush, which is a yeast infection of the mouth and throat.

After taking medicine, your child should always rinse their mouth with water and spit it out. This will help avoid thrush. Sometimes it is easier to have your child brush their teeth. For very young children, you might use a clean wet washcloth to gently wipe the inside of your child's cheeks.

You should wash your child's face after giving ICSs with a nebulizer and mask.

Your child might grow more slowly during the first year of using ICSs. In some cases this can affect your child's adult height. Your doctor should measure your child's height at least every 6 months while on treatment. Asthma that **isn't** controlled can also slow down growth.

ICSs are **not** the same as steroids used to build muscles.

What should I keep in mind?

- Inhaled corticosteroids are the best controller medicine.
- You can give ICSs with a metered-dose inhaler and a holding chamber, a dry powder inhaler, or a nebulizer.
- Your child takes ICSs every day, even when they have **no** signs of asthma.
- An ICS **doesn't** stop an asthma attack. You'll need quick-relief medicine for an asthma attack. Make sure you always have quick-relief medicine handy.

Controller Medicine – Inhaled Corticosteroids

What can I do at home?

- Know how to use a:
  - Metered-dose inhaler.
  - Holding chamber with a metered-dose inhaler.
  - Nebulizer machine. (See "Using a Nebulizer," page 91.)

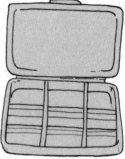

- Teach other members of the family how to use inhalers.

- Have a daily routine for your child to take their medicine. Give your child their medicine at the same time every day. This way you **won't** forget. And your child will learn when it's time to take the medicine.

- Have your child take ICSs after breakfast, before brushing teeth. Take again at bedtime, before brushing teeth. There are some free inhaler reminder apps you can get for your cell phone to help you remember.

- **Don't** nag your child to take their medicine. Be gentle but firm. Be matter-of-fact about taking medicine. Your child will learn "this is the way it is."

- Store medicines in a plastic box. **Don't** keep them in the bathroom or near water. Water makes the medicine powder cake into a hard ball.
  - Store metered-dose inhalers and holding chambers with the cap on.
  - Keep them in a cool, dry place.
  - Store medicine out of the reach of young children.

When do I call the doctor or nurse?

- Call when you **don't** understand what your doctor told you to do about your child's medicine.

- Call anytime you **can't** give your child the medicine in the Asthma Action Plan.

- Call and tell the doctor when your child has bad side effects from the medicine.

- Call when you need a refill of the medicine.

Other Controller Medicines

What is it?

Your child takes controller medicines every day, even with **no** signs of asthma. This section tells about controller medicines that **aren't** inhaled corticosteroids.

What should I know?

Controller medicines listed below can help, but they're **not** the first choice. They might **not** work as well as inhaled corticosteroids.

Leukotriene (loo-ko-treen) modifiers

These are pills your child can swallow. For young children, this medicine comes as a chewable pill or a powder you can sprinkle on food.

- Leukotriene modifiers are usually used for mild asthma. It is more common to use them when your child also has allergies.
- You can use them in children age 12 months and older.
- They're easy to give young children because you can take them by mouth.
- These medicines help prevent asthma signs. They also relieve nasal (nose) problems.
- These medicines are sometimes given **even if your child is also on** an inhaled corticosteroid.

Here are some leukotriene modifiers:

- Singulair® (montelukast)
- Accolate® (zafirlukast)

Here are some possible side effects:

- Headache
- Dizziness
- Rash
- Upset stomach
- Nightmares
- Aggressive behavior
- Worsening depression

Long-acting beta agonists (LABAs)

These medicines relax the airway muscle, keeping the airway open. A LABA comes as a metered-dose inhaler or a dry powder inhaler.

- A LABA works for up to 12 hours. You might hear this medicine called "long acting."
- Because LABAs are long acting, they can prevent asthma signs at night.
- Kids with asthma should never be given a daily LABA for asthma control unless it is mixed with an ICS. The only time it might be used by itself is to prevent asthma signs caused by exercise.
- This medicine is **not** approved for children less than 4 years old.
- You **must** give LABAs **with** an inhaled corticosteroid.
- **Never** use LABAs to treat an asthma attack.

- **Never** take LABAs more than 2 times a day.
- **Never** give more of this medicine than what is ordered.

Here are some long-acting beta agonists:

- Serevent® (salmeterol)
- Foradil® (formoterol)

Here are some possible side effects:

- Shakiness
- Fast heart rate
- Muscle cramps
- Headache

A LABA often comes together with an inhaled corticosteroid as 1 medicine.

- Salmeterol and fluticasone come together as Advair®.
- Formoterol and budesonide come together as Symbicort®.
- Formoterol and mometasone come together as Dulera®

Theophylline

Theophylline is a controller medicine that **isn't** used often. It comes as syrup, pill, or shot.

- Theophylline can work in the body for 8-24 hours.
- It's sometimes given to control asthma signs at night.

Here are some kinds of theophylline:

- Slobid®
- Theo-Dur®
- Uniphyl®

This medicine can cause these bad side effects:

- Upset stomach
- Throwing up
- Fast heart beat
- Shaking
- Seizures

Call your doctor right away to report a bad side effect. The doctor will need to do blood tests to check how much theophylline is in the blood.

What should I keep in mind?

- Your child takes controller medicine every day even when they have **no** asthma signs.
- Controller medicine works by preventing asthma signs.
- Some kids need to be on more than one controller medication.

What should I do at home?

- Know these things about the medicine you're giving your child:
  - Name of the medicine
  - What the medicine looks like
  - What time to give the medicine
  - How much of the medicine to give
  - How to give the medicine
  - What the side effects are
- Follow your child's Asthma Action Plan.

- Watch for side effects. Report side effects to your doctor.

- Keep a supply of your child's medicines on hand. Get refills when needed.

When do I call the doctor or nurse?

- Call the doctor if your child has bad side effects from the medicine.

- Call if your child's asthma is worse.

Oral Steroids

What is it?

Oral steroids are medicines that treat inflamed airways. Your child swallows them for a severe asthma attack.

What should I know?

Steroids that your child swallows are very good at stopping an asthma attack. But they are **not** the first choice for controlling asthma in children. To control asthma, it's best to use steroids that your child inhales. The right ICS, given properly, works very well to keep asthma attacks away.

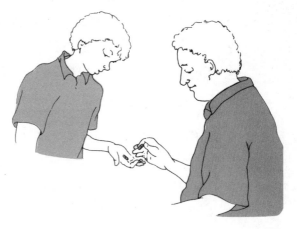

- When you use them right away, oral steroids can stop inflammation quickly. They might take 6-8 hours to start working.

- You might give oral steroids for 5-7 days.

- The doctor will order the lowest dose for the shortest period of time possible. It is best to use only what it takes to get asthma under control. This helps decrease side effects.

- Your child might need oral steroids for a long time if controller medicine **isn't** working.

- Sometimes the doctor might tell you to "taper" the dose. This means you give less and less medicine every day until you stop giving it.

- A good goal of treatment is to be on the right ICS controller at the right dose so you **don't** need to give your child oral steroids very often.

- This **isn't** the same steroid that's used to build muscles.

Here are some oral steroids:

- Prednisone® (prednisone)
- Prelone® and Orapred® (prednisolone)
- Medrol® (prednisolone)
- Decadron® (dexamethasone)

Your child might have some side effects when taking oral steroids for 5-7 days. These might include:

- Eating more food.
- Feeling hyper, or having trouble settling down.
- Trouble sleeping.

Side effects when using oral steroids for weeks or months might include:

- Puffiness or weight gain.
- Slowed growth.
- High blood pressure.
- Weak bones.
- Eye problems.
- Acne rash.
- Stomach problems.

Oral Steroids

Oral steroids might be part of the Asthma Action Plan if your child has bad attacks.

What should I keep in mind?

- Oral steroids are very strong medicines usually used to stop an asthma attack.

- Oral steroids might prevent an emergency room visit. Your child's doctor might ask you to give your child a dose of oral steroid while on your way to the emergency room. If your doctor wants you to do this, ask to have it on the written Asthma Action Plan.

- You might need oral steroids for a longer time for bad cases of asthma.

- There can be bad side effects if your child takes oral steroids for weeks or months.

What can I do at home?

- Make sure you're giving the right dose of oral steroids.

- Make sure you give it for the number of days the doctor told you.

- Give oral steroids in the morning, so your child **doesn't** have trouble going to sleep.

- Tell every doctor your child sees that your child is taking oral steroids for asthma.

When do I call the doctor or nurse?

- Call when you start using oral steroids as a part of your Asthma Action Plan.

- Call to schedule a visit to the doctor after starting oral steroids.

- Tell the doctor when your child has used oral steroids several times during the year.

Helping Your Child Take Medicines

5

Notes

_____

_____

_____

_____

_____

_____

_____

_____

_____

_____

_____

_____

_____

_____

_____

Metered-Dose Inhalers with Holding Chambers

What is it?

A metered-dose inhaler is a small tool with medicine inside. You press down on it to get a mist of medicine. Your child breathes the medicine in through their mouth. You can use an inhaler with either controller medicine or quick-relief medicine.

What should I know?

Medicine your child breathes in works better than medicine they swallow. Medicine goes straight into the lungs when your child breathes it in. There are also fewer side effects from the medicine, and it works quicker.

A metered-dose inhaler:

- Holds the medicine.
- Has a gas that sprays the medicine out of the can.
- Is a pressurized can. That means the medicine is squeezed tight inside.
- Has a meter that gives your child the right dose of medicine with each puff.
- Can travel with you when you leave home.

It's very important that you know how to use the metered-dose inhaler. You can ask the pharmacist, nurse, or doctor to show you.

Metered-Dose Inhalers with Holding Chambers

If your child needs quick-relief at the same time the controller is due, always use the quick-relief inhaler first. This will open the lungs for the controller medicine. Wait 2 minutes before using the other inhaler.

All kids should always use a holding chamber to help get the full dose of medicine. (See "Using a Holding Chamber," page 82.)

How to use a metered-dose inhaler:

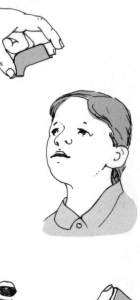

- Always follow the instructions that come with your inhaler. They are on a piece of paper, folded inside the box with the inhaler.

- Most metered-dose inhalers need to be primed. This means you need to get the can ready to give to your child. You will need to prime it the first time you open a new inhaler before you give it to your child. Usually the first time you use your new inhaler it is primed by 4 puffs. You need to prime it again every time it has **not** been used for 2 weeks or more. You will also need to prime it again if the inhaler drops to the floor.

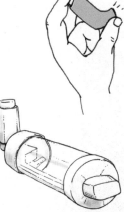

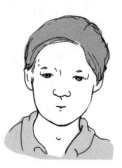

- Before you begin, wash your hands. Most inhalers have "dose-counter" numbers on the plastic case so you can see how many "puffs" are in the can when it's full. You can also look at the number to see how many puffs are left in the can after using it. Look at the inhaler to see what that number is. The number can be found on the opposite side of the mouthpiece.

To prime your child's inhaler

1. Hold the inhaler in one hand. Shake it hard while you count slowly to 5.

2. Hold the inhaler so it does **not** point at you or anyone's face.

3. Press the top of the can. You should hear a soft blowing sound.

4. Shake hard again while counting to 5. Press the top of the can down while keeping it pointed away from anyone's face.

5. Follow the steps again, in order, 2 more times.

6. Look at the dose-counter number on the can. It should have 4 less puffs in it than when you took it out of the box.

7. The medicine is now ready to use.

To give your child ICSs with an inhaler

1. Wash your hands. Wash your child's hands.

2. Remove the cap. Make sure there's nothing inside the mouthpiece that shouldn't be there.

3. Insert the mouthpiece into the rubber opening at the end of the holding chamber. It should fit well and **not** be loose.

4. You or your child should hold the inhaler upright. Put your pointer finger on top of the inhaler, or help your child do this. Put your or your child's thumb on the bottom of the inhaler.

5. Shake the inhaler hard like you did to prime it. You will need to shake it like that before every puff. It's important to mix the medication like this so you are always giving the right dose.

6. Tilt your child's head up. Have them open their mouth. Have them breathe out. Put the holding chamber into your child's mouth so it is behind the teeth and on top of the tongue. Have your child bite down gently to make sure it stays put. Have your child keep their lips tight around the mouthpiece.

7. You or your child should press down 1 time on top of the inhaler. Have your child breathe in slowly. Some holding chambers make a whistling sound if your child breathes in too fast. The goal is to **not** hear that sound. The medicine works best if you breathe it in slowly. If your child has trouble, have them practice using the holding chamber without medicine.

8. Have your child hold their breath for 10 seconds. (Count to 10.)

9. Tell your child to breathe out slowly.

10. Put the cap back on the mouthpiece. This will keep it clean and ready to use.

11. Wait 1 minute before your child takes another dose if needed.

12. Have your child rinse out their mouth and spit.

To give your child ICSs with a mask

Younger children should use a holding chamber with a mask. Some older kids do better with a mask, too. If your child has a holding chamber with a mask:

1. Follow the above directions for priming and shaking until you have finished step 4.

2. Put the mask with the holding chamber on your child's face so that it covers the mouth and nose. Press it gently against the face so the medicine **won't** leak out of it.

3. Keep the holding chamber mask gently pressed on to the face with one hand. Use the other hand to hold the inhaler. Put your pointer finger on the top of it, and your thumb on the bottom.

4. Press 1 time.

5. Have your child take 6-10 slow deep breaths. Some holding chambers have a little flap that moves as the child breathes. You can count how many times it moves in and out. You can also count how many times your child takes in a breath. Watch the child's chest and count the number of breaths.

6. Remember, the holding chamber should **not** make any whistling or squealing noises. If it does, have your child breathe in more slowly.

7. Have your child brush their teeth, or rinse and spit with water.

8. Gently wash your child's face to rinse off the medicine.

What should I keep in mind?

- Inhaled medicines work better than medicine you swallow.
- Your child will have fewer side effects with inhaled medicine.
- You must use the metered dose inhaler correctly for the medicine to get into the lungs.
- A holding chamber is very important to help your child breathe in all of the medicine dose. This is especially important if your child:
  - Is small.
  - Has trouble using an inhaler.
  - Is taking inhaled corticosteroids.

Metered-Dose Inhalers with Holding Chambers

- Ask your doctor for a holding chamber.
  - The best kinds (valved holding chambers) have a valve so the medicine stays in the chamber until your child inhales it.
  - You should also make sure the one your doctor gives you is a non-electrostatic (ee-**leck**-tro-**stah**-tick) holding chamber. That helps make sure the medicine **doesn't** stick to the inside of the holding chamber.
- Experts say you should use the holding chamber for all metered dose inhalers whenever possible. You **must** use the holding chamber for the metered-dose inhaler controller medicines.
- Most doctors give kids metered-dose inhalers that need holding chambers. Some inhalers are filled with medicine that is a special dry powder instead of liquid. Dry powder inhalers (DPIs) must **not** be used with holding chambers and do **not** need shaking.
- Make sure you know what type of inhaler your doctor has ordered for your child. Make sure you understand how to use it.

What can I do at home?

- Learn all about the inhaler your child is going to use.
- Watch to make sure your child uses the inhaler the right way.
- Keep track of how much medicine is in the metered-dose inhaler. Here are some tips:
  - Ask your pharmacist when you will need a refill.
  - Write the date on the inhaler.

Metered-Dose Inhalers with Holding Chambers

- Use a paper calendar to remind you when you'll need a new inhaler. You can also use your cell phone to set a reminder in your calendar a week before it is due.

- Some pharmacies can set up reminders for you. They will call you to ask if you want a refill before it's due. Ask your pharmacy if you would like to have them call you with reminders.

- Check the dose counter number on the back of the inhaler. When the numbers turn red, call the pharmacy right away for a refill.

- If you **don't** have an inhaler with a dose counter, ask the pharmacist how many puffs are in the inhaler.

- Divide this by the number of times a day you use the inhaler. This will tell you how many days the inhaler will last. You can ask your doctor or pharmacist for help figuring this out. Mark the date on your calendar.

- **Don't** use an inhaler when your child has already taken all the doses. Your child **won't** get the right dose of medicine.

- An empty metered-dose inhaler might still sound like it has medicine in it when you shake it. If the dose-counter number is on "0", there is no more medicine in the inhaler. The special liquid that stays behind is **not** medicine. It is what helps the medicine spray out of the can when you press it.

- Get a new inhaler if you're **not** sure the inhaler still has medicine in it.

- Get a new inhaler if it has been opened for more than 6 months.

- Ask the doctor for a prescription for 2 inhalers. Before the first one is empty, get a refill.

How to take care of your child's inhalers

Metered-dose inhalers sometimes get clogged. Different types of metered-dose inhalers need different care. Read the instructions that come with them in the box. Ask your pharmacist to help you find the directions the first time.

- Metered-dose inhalers with quick-relief medicines
  - After each use, wipe the mouthpiece with a tissue.
  - The plastic case should be washed once a week during the times your child needs it to help with signs of asthma. You must **never** let the medicine can get wet.
  - Gently pull the can out of the plastic case and put it somewhere safe and dry. Choose a place you **won't** forget.
  - Run warm water through the plastic case for about 30 seconds. Shake the extra water out of it.
  - Let it dry. When it is completely dry, replace the can back in the plastic holder.
  - Cleaning will help to keep the quick-relief inhaler free of clogs.
  - Store the inhaler upright in a clean plastic bag.
- Metered-dose inhalers with ICS controller medicines
  - After each use, wipe the mouthpiece with a tissue.
  - Once a week or so, use a cotton swab to clean the tiny hole deep inside the mouthpiece.
  - **Don't** take the container apart or clean it with water.

- Put the cap on it and store it upright in a clean plastic bag.
- All inhalers
  - Always keep the inhalers in the same place so you can find them when you need them.
  - Keep the inhalers out of reach of small children.
  - Take your inhalers with you each time you go to the doctor.

When do I call the doctor or nurse?

- Call the doctor when you need a prescription for an inhaler.
- Call if you're **not** sure how to use or care for the inhaler.
- Call if you **don't** feel the inhaler is helping your child's asthma signs.
- Call if you need help knowing how many days the inhaler will last.
- Call the doctor if your child's asthma is getting worse.

Using a Holding Chamber

What is it?

A holding chamber is a plastic tube you put on an inhaler.
It helps your child get the full dose of the medicine.
You can use it with a mask or mouthpiece.

What should I know?

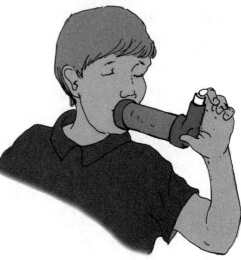

You place a holding chamber between the inhaler and your child's mouth. It's often called a "spacer," but a holding chamber has a special valve so the medicine does **not** leak out easily. Spacers are old fashioned. They do **not** have a special valve. Make sure you have a holding chamber that is **not** electrostatic.

A holding chamber helps get more medicine into the lungs. All children should use one for their metered-dose inhalers. It will help make sure your child gets the full dose.

A holding chamber:

- Keeps medicine from going into the air around your child's mouth and face.

- Holds the medicine to give your child time to breathe it in slowly and deeply.
- Keeps medicine from hitting the back of the throat. The medicine goes straight into the lungs.

How to use a holding chamber with an inhaler

Always follow the directions that come in the package.

- Wash your hands. Wash your child's hands.
- Remove the cap from the inhaler.
- Put the mouthpiece into the end of the holding chamber.

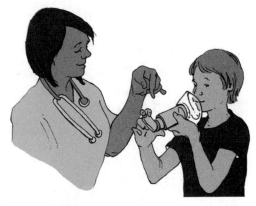

- Shake the inhaler with the holding chamber for 5 full seconds.

Have your child follow these steps:

1. Stand or sit up as straight as you can.

2. Breathe out.

3. Use one hand to hold the holding chamber and the other hand for the inhaler. Hold the inhaler with your pointer finger on top and your thumb below.

4. Place the mouthpiece behind the teeth and on top of the tongue.

5. Close your lips tight around the mouthpiece.

6. Push down the top of the inhaler once.

7. Take a slow, deep breath in.

8. If you hear a squeal or whistle from the holding chamber, ask your child to breathe in more slowly.

9. Hold your breath for 10 seconds. (Count to 10 in your head.)

10. Remove the mouthpiece and breathe normally.

11. Most times, your doctor will want your child to take 2 puffs of medicine. If you need a second puff, wait 1 minute. Then repeat steps 4 to 10.

12. Put the cap back on the mouthpiece.

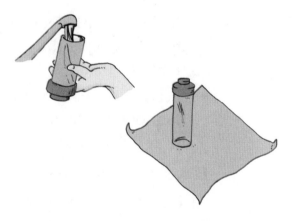

When you are using an inhaler with a small child:

- Hold the child on your lap. You can also sit or stand behind the child.

- Reach around to help the child.

- When a child **can't** hold their breath, use 6-10 normal breaths as a count.

How to clean the holding chamber

Clean the holding chamber once a week. Always clean it the way the directions tell you to. Most holding chambers **can't** go in the dishwasher.

1. Take the holding chamber apart.

2. Soak it in warm water. Use a little dish soap. Soak for 10 minutes.

3. Rinse with clear water.

4. Shake off any extra water.

5. Place holding chamber parts on a paper towel to dry. **Don't** rub them dry or scrub the inside of the chamber.

Get a new holding chamber when:
- The holding chamber is cracked.
- Rubber parts are hard, curled, or cracked.
- Any part is broken.
- Any part is missing.

What should I keep in mind?
- A holding chamber will make sure your child gets the full dose of medicine.
- All children should use a holding chamber.
- Babies and young children will need a mask and a holding chamber.
- One push on the top of the inhaler is one puff. Most children get 2 puffs of medicine for their full dose.
- When a child **can't** hold their breath, let them breathe 6 normal breaths for each dose.

What can I do at home?
- Learn how to use the inhaler with the holding chamber. Make sure your child is using it the right way. If not, they **won't** get the full dose of medicine.

- Ask your pharmacist to show you how to give your child the medicine. Ask if they can show you pictures or videos about how to use the inhaler and holding chamber.

- Keep everything in one place and ready to use.

- Keep the holding chamber clean.

- When your child's holding chamber is worn or broken, get a new one.

- **Never** let a child use another child's holding chamber or inhaler.

- Make follow-up doctor appointments. Keep doctor appointments.

When do I call the doctor or nurse?

- Call if you need help learning to use the inhaler with the holding chamber. Ask the doctor or nurse to show you how. They might have pictures or videos to help you. Have your child show the doctor they can use the metered-dose inhaler with the holding chamber.

- Call the doctor when you **don't** think your child is getting the full dose of medicine.

Using a Mask with Holding Chamber

What is it?

A mask fits over a child's nose and mouth. It helps very young children get a full dose of inhaler medicine.

What should I know?

Children under 5 years old might need to use a holding chamber with a mask when taking inhaler medicine.

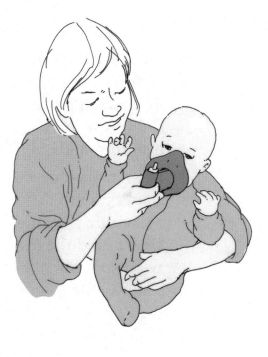

- A holding chamber is a tube between the inhaler and a mask.

- The mask fits onto the holding chamber.

- The mask covers the child's mouth and nose. The mask makes a seal so the medicine **can't** leak out. The medicine goes through the mouth and nose into the lungs.

- The mask must fit **tightly** around your child's mouth and nose. It **shouldn't** go above the bridge of the nose into the eyes. It **shouldn't** go under the chin, either.

How to use a holding chamber and mask with an inhaler

Always follow the directions in the package with the inhaler, holding chamber, and mask.

- Wash your hands. Wash your child's hands.

- Have your child sit up.

- Remove the cap from the inhaler.

- Put the inhaler into one end of the holding chamber.

- Put the mask at the other end of the holding chamber.

- Shake for 5 seconds.

- Hold small children on your lap. You can also sit or stand behind the child. Reach around to help the child.

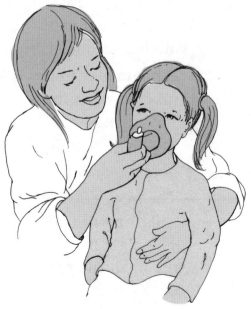

- Put the mask over your child's mouth and nose. Make sure it's snug. **Don't** hold the mask away from the mouth and nose. If you do, you **won't** give the full dose of medicine.

- Use one hand to hold the holding chamber. Use the pointer finger and thumb of your other hand to hold the inhaler.

- Push the top of the inhaler once.

Using a Mask with Holding Chamber

- Have your child take 6 normal breaths. Or leave the mask on and have your child breathe normally for 20-30 seconds.

- Remove the mask and have your child breathe normally. **Don't** remove it until your child has breathed in the medicine.

- Wait 1 minute before giving another puff. Only give another puff if the doctor tells you. One press down on the inhaler is 1 puff.

- Put the cap back on the mouthpiece.

- Wash your child's face with warm soapy water. Rinse your child's mouth with water.

- Rinse the mask with water. Let it air dry.

What should I keep in mind?

A face mask helps a baby or small child get the right dose of medicine.

What can I do at home?

- Ask the doctor or pharmacist what mask will work best for your child. Masks come in sizes for babies, young children, and adults. Some masks for children come in different colors.

- Have your child use the mask. Let your child play with the mask. Let them put the mask on a favorite toy, like a teddy bear or doll. Put it on yourself to show them how it fits. Doing these things will help your child feel less afraid.

- Make a game of using the mask. Sing to your child.

Using a Mask with Holding Chamber

- Put on your child's favorite TV show while using the mask.

- Make sure the mask fits snugly over your child's mouth and nose. Make sure it's **not** in the eyes.

- Learn how to use the inhaler with the holding chamber and a mask. Ask the pharmacist to show you. Ask if they have pictures or a video of how to use the mask, holding chamber, and inhaler.

- You can also look at some websites. Ask your doctor which ones will give you the right information.

- Wash the mask every day in warm, soapy water. Put it on a towel to air dry.

- Keep everything you use in one place and ready to use.

- Know when you need a new inhaler. Have a new inhaler ready to use.

- Make follow-up doctor appointments. Keep doctor appointments.

When do I call the doctor or nurse?

- Call if you need them to show you how to give medicine to your child. Ask if they can show you pictures or a video of how to use the mask, holding chamber, and inhaler.

- Call if you're having trouble using the inhaler with the holding chamber and mask.

- Call when you need a refill for an inhaler.

Using a Nebulizer

What is it?

A nebulizer is a machine. It mixes air with a liquid medicine to make a mist. Your child breathes this mist into their lungs.

What should I know?

- You can use a nebulizer to give both quick-relief and controller medicines.
- It takes about 10 minutes to give medicine to a child with a nebulizer.
- The best asthma nebulizers are called "jet" nebulizers.
- Most nebulizer machines have to be plugged in. Some run on batteries. Some machines can be plugged into a cigarette lighter in the car.

You can use a nebulizer:

- With very young children who have trouble using a metered-dose inhaler.
- When a child is having an asthma attack.
- When a child has bad asthma.

How to use a nebulizer

Always follow the directions that come with your nebulizer.

Get ready:

1. Place the nebulizer machine on a table. Put it in reach of an electric outlet. Put it where you can reach the off/on switch. Put it where it's safe.

2. Plug the machine into the electric outlet.

3. Wash your hands. Wash your child's hands.

4. Make sure your child is comfortable. If they're in diapers, make sure the diaper is dry. It's better **not** to use the nebulizer when a child is fussy or crying.

5. Have something for your child to do. Give them a book, a toy, or a doll.

6. Most medicines for nebulizers come already mixed in the dose your child takes. For others you might need to measure the dose. Put it in the nebulizer cup. Screw or click the cap on tightly.

7. Attach the top of the nebulizer cup to the mask or mouthpiece.

8. Attach tubing to the machine and to the nebulizer cup.

9. Turn the nebulizer on.

Give the medicine:

1. Make sure a mist is coming through the mask or mouthpiece.

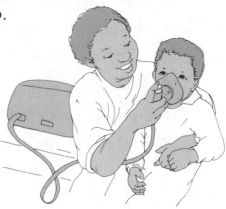

2. Sit in a chair and hold your child. An older child might sit alone in a chair.

3. **If using a mask:** Place the mask over your child's mouth and nose. Make sure it fits snugly around the mouth and nose. Make sure it **doesn't** go into the eyes. **Don't** hold the mask away from the mouth and nose. Your child **won't** get the full dose of medicine.
   If using a mouthpiece: Place it between the child's teeth and seal their lips tightly around it.

4. Have your child hold their head up and take slow and deep breaths through the mouth. Have them keep breathing until the medicine is gone.

5. Stop if your child throws up or has a coughing spell. Turn off the machine. Let your child rest a few minutes. Then start the nebulizer again.

6. Turn the machine off when the medicine is gone.

7. Have your child take some deep breaths. They might need to cough or use a tissue.

8. Wash your hands with warm water and soap.

9. Have your child wash their hands.

10. Have your child rinse their mouth with water and spit it out. This will remove any medicine from the mouth.

11. Wash or wipe off your child's face.

Caring for the machine

Follow the directions that come with the machine. **Not** all nebulizers can be cleaned the same way. Always unplug the machine before cleaning it.

After each use:

- Rinse the nebulizer cup with warm water. Let it dry.
- Throw the cup away if it's meant to be used only once.
- Wipe the machine with a clean, damp cloth.

At the end of every day:

- Wash the cup, mask, and mouthpiece in warm, soapy water. Use dish soap. Shake to remove any water.
- Place the pieces on a paper towel to air dry. Or put them back on the machine. Turn the machine on for a few minutes, and the pieces will dry quickly.
- Cover the machine with a clean cloth. **Don't** store the machine on the floor.

Every 3 days:

- Clean the machine:
  - Use the cleaning mixture listed in the machine's directions.
  - Or use a vinegar solution of ½ cup white vinegar and 1½ cups water. Soak for 1 hour. Rinse with water under the faucet. Shake off the water. Place the parts on a paper towel to dry.
- Make sure the tubing and mask are dry before placing them in a plastic bag.

Every 6 months:

- Replace the cup and the tubing.

- Change the filter. Or change the filter when the directions tell you to.

What should I keep in mind?

- A nebulizer is the best way to give medicine to a very young child. The best time to give the treatment is when your child is quiet or sleeping. When a child is fussy, wait a while before using the nebulizer.

- Use a nebulizer if your child has trouble using a metered-dose inhaler.

- A nebulizer is the best way to give your child medicine when they are having an asthma attack.

- You must use the machine the right way for your child to get the full dose of medicine.

- You must use a special mask for ICSs used in a nebulizer. Check with your doctor or pharmacist to be sure you have the right mask.

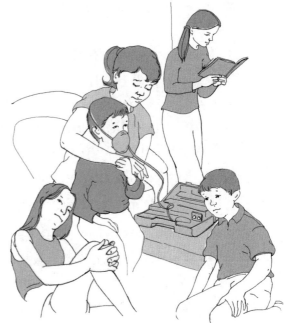

- If your child has the special mask for nebulizer ICSs, it is OK to use the same mask for quick-relief medicine.

- **Don't** hold the mask out from the face. If you do, your child **won't** get the medicine. The mask must be snug around the nose and mouth. Make sure it's **not** over the eyes.
- Ask the person who brings the nebulizer to your home to show you how to use it.
- Here are some things to do with your child while they use the nebulizer:
    - Hold the child in your lap.
    - Use this as a time with all your children. Have them all sit with you.
    - Read a story.
    - Sing to your child.
    - Let your child watch a favorite cartoon.

What can I do at home?

- Keep all of the papers and directions that came with the nebulizer. Store them where you can find them. Look for the phone number to call when the machine **isn't** working. Keep that phone number handy.
- Let your baby or toddler play with the mask.
- Check all the tubes anytime the machine **isn't** working.
- Make sure they're on tight and **not** twisted.
- Keep the machine clean. This will keep your child from getting sick with an infection.
- Store medicine in a cool and dry place. Throw away medicine that changes color or has crystals.
- Always keep an extra nebulizer cup and mask in case you need it.

When do I call the doctor or nurse?

- Call anytime you **can't** give medicine with the nebulizer.

- Call if your nebulizer **isn't** working, and you **don't** know what to do for your child.

- Call if you think the medicine **isn't** helping your child.

Dry Powder Inhalers

What is it?

A dry powder inhaler holds a fine powder medicine. Your child breathes the medicine in.

What should I know?

The inhaler holds the dry powder medicine. You can use a dry powder inhaler for both quick-relief and controller medicines. Some children as young as 4 years can use a dry powder inhaler. It works like this:

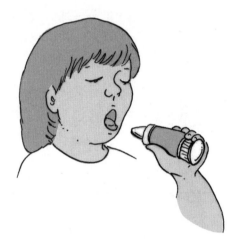

- Your child holds the inhaler in their hand.
- They place the inhaler in their mouth.
- Your child breathes in deeply and quickly.
- The air carries the medicine into the lungs.
- The right dose of medicine goes into the lungs.

Dry powder inhalers are small. You can take them with you anywhere. They come in many shapes and sizes. You **don't** need to use a holding chamber or mask. And you **don't** need to shake or prime the inhaler.

There are 4 types of dry powder inhalers:

Multidose tube inhaler

- Pulmicort Flexhaler® (budesonide)
- Asmanex Twisthaler® (mometasone)

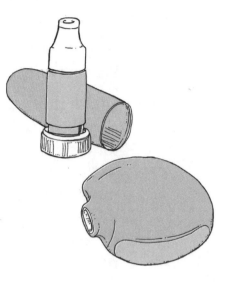

Single dose tube inhaler

- Foradil® (formoterol) Dry powder disk inhaler.

Dry powder disk inhaler

- Flovent Diskus® (fluticasone)
- Advair Diskus® (fluticasone/salmeterol)

Breath actuated multidose inhaler

- Arnuity® Ellipta® (fluticasone furoate)
- ProAir® RespiClick (albuterol)

It's very important that you know how to use the inhaler. You can ask the pharmacist, nurse, or doctor to show you and your child how.

Some inhalers come with medicine inside them. With others, you put the medicine in right before you use it. You have to put the medicine into a single dose inhaler each time you use it.

Dry Powder Inhalers

How to use a dry powder inhaler with kids 4 years of age and older:

Always follow any directions that come with your inhaler.

1. Wash your hands. Wash your child's hands.

2. Check the mouthpiece for dirt or dry medicine. Wipe it clean if you need to.

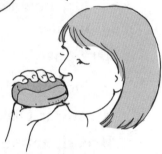

3. Have your child breathe out as much air as they can.

4. Keeping the inhaler flat, follow the directions to trigger it.

5. Have your child breathe in fast and deep. This will pull the powder into the lungs. Have your child hold their breath for 10 seconds. (Count to 10.)

6. Take away the inhaler.

7. Have your child breathe normally.

8. Wait 10 seconds before giving a second dose if needed.

9. Put the cap back on the mouthpiece.

Dry Powder Inhalers

What should I keep in mind?

- The dry powder inhaler must be used the right way to get the full dose of medicine.
- There's **no** need to shake or prime the inhaler before you use it.
- To use the inhaler, tell your child:
  - Breathe out.
  - Put the inhaler in your mouth.
  - Take a fast, deep breath. Hold your breath for 10 seconds.
- The medicine goes into the lungs when the child takes in a deep breath.
- Always hold the dry powder inhaler flat, **not** upright.
- You must **not** use a holding chamber with a dry powder inhaler.

What can I do at home?

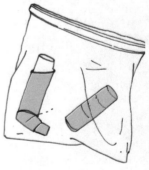

- Make sure your child knows how to use the inhaler.
- Keep track of how much medicine is in the inhaler.
  - Some inhalers count the doses. This makes it easy to know how many are left.
  - Ask the pharmacist how long the inhaler will last for your child.
- Get refills **before** your child's inhaler is empty.
- If your child uses more than one inhaler, label them. Then you'll know which one to use and when.

- Watch to make sure your child is using the inhaler the right way. You might have to help them.

- Store the inhaler in a clean, plastic bag. Keep it in a cool, dry place. **Don't** store it in a damp place like the bathroom. Dampness can make the medicine clump into a ball.

- Wipe the mouthpiece clean. **Don't** wash your dry powder inhaler.

- **Don't** use the inhaler after the "use before" or expiration date on the package.

- Take your child's inhaler and all medicines with you when you go to the doctor.

When do I call a doctor or nurse?

- Call if you're **not** sure how to use the inhaler.

- Call if the inhaler **isn't** helping your child's asthma signs.

- Call when you need a prescription for a new inhaler.

Your Child's Health 6

Notes

_____

_____

_____

_____

_____

_____

_____

_____

_____

_____

_____

_____

_____

_____

_____

Benefits of Exercise

What is it?

Exercise is good for your child. It's important to make the lungs strong. It can make your child's asthma better.

What should I know?

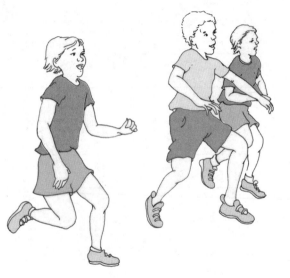

- Your child needs to exercise. Exercise builds muscles. Exercise helps lungs grow. Exercise makes your child feel good and helps with weight control.

- Exercise is part of your plan to care for your child. It will help your child do all the things other children do.

- **Don't** let your child exercise when they're having asthma signs.

- Exercise can be an asthma trigger. (See "When Exercise Brings on Asthma," page 108.)

- You can take control of your child's asthma so your child can exercise.

- Here are some important ways that exercise helps your child:
  - Your child can do what other children do.
  - Exercise helps your child stay well.
  - Your child **won't** miss school.
  - You child can have a normal life.
  - Your child might need less medicine.
  - Your child **won't** have to go to the emergency room a lot.
- Your child should exercise 5 days a week, for 60 minutes.
- The doctor might tell you to give albuterol before exercise. This will prevent signs of asthma.
- Your child should have **no** signs of asthma before starting to exercise.
- Your child **shouldn't** exercise outside if there's something in the air, like smog or smoke.
- Your child should do warm-ups before exercise. Stretches, jogging, and short sprints are all good.

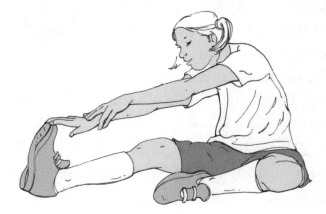

What should I keep in mind?

- Your child needs to exercise. Exercise builds muscles. Exercise helps the lungs grow. Exercise makes your child feel good.
- Exercise is a part of the plan to care for your child.
- Exercise will help your child do all the things other children do.
- You can take charge of your child's asthma so your child can exercise.

What can I do at home?

- Make sure your child can breathe through the nose. It's important to keep the mouth shut so air goes through the nose. This will warm and moisten the air. Help your child blow their nose and keep it clean.

- Teach your child to breathe through the nose while doing exercise.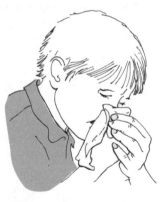

- **Don't** let your child start exercising if they're coughing or wheezing. They shouldn't have any mucus or rattling, either.

- **Don't** let your child exercise outdoors when there's a lot of smog. **Don't** let them exercise outdoors when it's very cold or very hot, either. Find someplace inside where your child can exercise.

- Have a plan for your child to exercise all year.
- Talk to your child's teachers about exercise for your child.

- Have a plan for when your child goes someplace where they might exercise. Examples are parties, camping, field trips, parks, playgrounds, and gyms.

When do I call the doctor or nurse?

- Call to talk about exercise for your child. Ask:
  - How much exercise should my child do?
  - How can I help my child exercise?
- Call before your child joins a sports team.
- Call when your child has trouble doing exercise.
- Call if your child needs to stop doing exercise.
- Call if your child's exercise triggers an asthma attack.
- Call if you're doing everything the doctor said, and your child is **still** having trouble doing exercise.

When Exercise Brings on Asthma

What is it?

Sometimes doing exercise brings on the signs of asthma. This is called "exercise-induced asthma," or "EIA."

What should I know?

The doctor will tell you if your child has EIA.

With EIA, your child has asthma signs after exercising or playing hard for 5-10 minutes or longer. A child might also have signs of asthma after they stop exercising or playing. Asthma signs usually go away 30 minutes after exercise or playing has stopped.

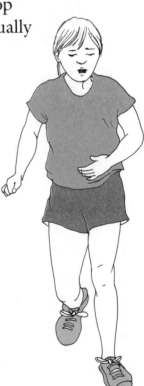

Here are some signs of EIA:

- Coughing
- Wheezing
- Chest pain or tightness
- Trouble catching their breath
- Feeling more tired than other kids
- Having asthma signs during hard exercise

Some things can make EIA worse. These things include:

- Cold weather.

- Dry air.
- Smog or smoke.
- Having a cold.
- Chemicals like chlorine from a pool.
- Pollen.

EIA happens because your child breathes differently during exercise:

- When **not** doing exercise, your child breathes through the nose. Air going through the nose gets moist (wet) before entering the lungs. This helps your child breathe.
- When doing exercise, your child breathes through an open mouth. This air is cool and dry. The cool, dry air makes the airway small and tight. This makes it harder for your child to breathe.

Some exercises are less likely than running to cause asthma signs. These exercises include:

- Walking.
- Riding a bike.
- Swimming.

Your doctor will tell you to give your child albuterol before exercise. Albuterol is a quick-relief medicine your child takes 5-15 minutes before exercise. It will prevent asthma signs for 3 hours.

- Keep an albuterol inhaler at home and at school. If your child uses a holding chamber, keep one at school, too.

- Make sure your child "warms up" before exercise. Some good warm-ups are stretching, walking, or a short run. Your child should warm up for 10-15 minutes.
- Make sure your child "cools down" after exercise, too. They should slow down and rest.

Exercise is important for **every** child, including children with asthma. Exercise helps keep a child healthy. Exercise makes a child feel good. Playing or doing sports is normal for a child.

Your doctor will help you plan exercise for your child.

What should I keep in mind?

- Every child needs to exercise.
- Take steps to help your child exercise.
- Visit a doctor to find out how to help your child exercise.
- Get a doctor's note saying it's OK for your child to have albuterol at school.
- EIA might occur alone. Or EIA might be part of poorly controlled asthma.

What can I do at home?

- Get your child to breathe through their nose.
- **Don't** have your child do hard exercise in cold weather.
- Have your child wear a face mask or a scarf over the mouth and nose in cold weather.
- Help your child find sports they can do. They might try volleyball, swimming, biking, walking, or baseball.

- Help your child exercise. Plan what your child can do. Give medicine as the doctor has told you to.

When do I call the doctor or nurse?

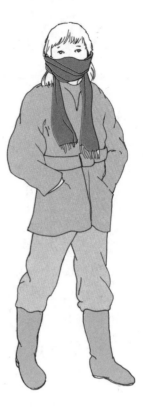

- See the doctor if you think your child has exercise-induced asthma.
- See the doctor if your child has to stop playing because they're having trouble breathing.
- See the doctor before your child joins a sports team.

Allergy Shots and Asthma

What is it?

An allergy shot gives your child a very small amount of what their body is allergic to. The shot will prevent the signs of allergy.

What should I know?

Many children who have asthma also have other allergic signs. Kids' allergies include:

- Hay fever.
- Skin rash.
- Insect stings.
- Food allergies. (Your doctor **doesn't** give shots for food allergies.)

An allergen is anything that gives your child an allergic reaction. Allergy shots lessen the symptoms caused by allergens.

An allergy shot contains a very small amount of what your child is allergic to. Here's an example: If your child is allergic to pollen, the shot will have a small amount of pollen.

- Allergy shots help your child's body block the allergen when it enters the body.
- Allergy shots help your child's body fight the allergen. Your child will have fewer signs like rash, sneezing, or wheezing.

- Doctors usually wait until a child is 5 years old before giving allergy shots.

- It usually takes 6 months or more before the allergy shots start helping.

- Children usually get allergy shots for 3-5 years.

When the shots work well, your doctor might tell you to give your child less asthma medicine. **Never stop giving medicine unless your child's doctor tells you to.**

Allergy shots might help when your child:

- Has asthma that's hard to control.

- Is allergic to allergens in the air.

- **Isn't** helped by asthma medicine or has side effects from the medicine.

- Has an allergic trigger that you **can't** take away.

- Is taking a lot of medicine for allergies.

- Has trouble taking medicine.

A special doctor usually gives allergy shots. This doctor is called an "allergy specialist."

- This doctor will do tests to find what your child is allergic to. The doctor will help you learn what's bothering your child.

- Allergies in children might **not** be the same as allergies in adults. The doctor will know what to do for your child.

Your child will get allergy shots in the doctor's office. Sometimes a child has a reaction to an allergy shot. The doctor will have your child wait 30 minutes before leaving the office after a shot. That way, if your child reacts to the shot, the doctor is there to help.

What should I keep in mind?

- Allergy shots can help a child have better control of their asthma.
- Allergy shots work best when you remove allergy triggers from your home.
- Allergy shots are for allergens in the air. Doctors **never** give allergy shots for a food allergy.
- Allergy shots can cost a lot of money. Ask your health insurance if they'll help pay for your child's allergy shots.
- If your child **doesn't** have health insurance, visit a community clinic. Ask for help getting insurance for your child.
- A child usually gets over their fear of shots when they see other children getting shots.

What can I do at home?

- Learn about how allergy shots can help your child.
- Talk to your child about going to the allergy specialist.

When do I call the doctor or nurse?

- Call to discuss if allergy shots will help your child.

Spit Up, Sour Stomach, and Heartburn

What is it?

Food and acid from the stomach can come back up the throat to your child's mouth. This can cause spit up, sour stomach, and heartburn.

What should I know?

When food and acid often flow back up from the stomach, it's a problem. The medical name for this problem is "acid reflux" or "GERD."

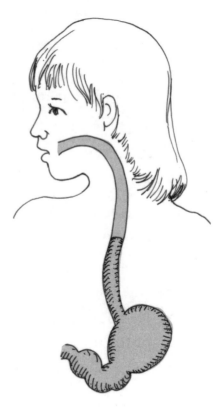

Acid reflux can cause trouble breathing. Food coming up from the stomach can get into the nose and lungs.

- Some spitting up is normal for babies.

- Acid reflux can happen when a young child lies down.

- Most babies and young children with acid reflux do better as they grow older.

Spit Up, Sour Stomach, and Heartburn

These are signs of an acid reflux problem in babies and young children:

- Always crying or fussy
- Always spitting up
- Bad breath
- Runny nose or drooling
- Croupy cough
- Spitting up 1 hour after eating
- Asthma signs often at night

These breathing problems can be signs of acid reflux, too:

- Wheezing
- Coughing at night
- Trouble sleeping
- Pneumonia
- Bronchitis

See a doctor to learn if your child has acid reflux. Your doctor will:

- Check your child.
- Ask questions to see if your child has acid reflux.
- Decide if your child has acid reflux or another health problem.
- Tell you what to do for your child.

Things that will help acid reflux in infants and young children:

- Keep the child sitting up for at least 45 minutes after eating. This helps keep food from coming back up the throat.
- Raise the head of the crib.
- Your doctor might tell you to change the baby's formula.
- Your doctor might tell you to change the times that you feed your baby.
- Your doctor might have you give your baby medicine.

Things that help acid reflux in an older child:

- Have the child eat small meals during the day.
- **Don't** let them eat 3 hours before going to bed.
- Try **not** to let them eat chocolate, garlic, onions, spicy foods, or fried foods.
- Try **not** to let them have soft drinks or drinks with caffeine.
- Raise the head of your child's bed about 6 inches. Put wood blocks under the legs.

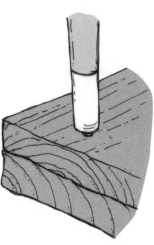

If these steps **don't** work, your doctor might have you give your child medicine.

What should I keep in mind?

- Problems with acid reflux can make asthma worse.
- You can help a child with acid reflux.

What can I do at home?

- Give your child any medicine the doctor has told you to give.
- Do what the doctor has told you to do for your child.
- Tell your whole family how to care for your child.

When do I call the doctor or nurse?

- Call if you think your child has acid reflux.
- Call when you run out of medicine to give your child.
- Call when you **don't** know what to do for your child.
- Call if your child **doesn't** get better.

Hay Fever

What is it?

Hay fever makes the inside of the nose pale, swollen, and watery. This happens when your child breathes in an allergen.

What should I know?

Problems with the nose make asthma worse. Hay fever can make it hard for your child to sleep. Your child might have ear problems or trouble doing well in school.

Doctors call hay fever "nasal allergy" or "allergic rhinitis."

Here are some signs that your child might have hay fever:

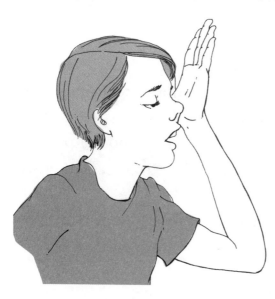

- Stuffy, runny, or itchy nose
- Always wiping or rubbing their nose
- Sneezing a lot
- Itchy, watery, red eyes
- Dark circles under the eyes
- Ear infections
- Coughing at night

Does your child have 2 or more of the signs above? Are you sure it's **not** a cold? Then it's probably hay fever.

Asthma triggers can also cause hay fever. (See "Asthma Triggers," page 18.)

The doctor will tell you if your child has hay fever. Your child's doctor will:

- Ask questions to see if your child has an allergy problem.
- Check your child.
- Give a chest x-ray, breathing test, or allergy test.
- Tell you if it's a nasal allergy, asthma, or another problem.
- Help you know what to do for your child.

Your doctor might have you give your child medicine. Antihistamine (an-ti-**his**-ti-meen) is a medicine that stops itching and sneezing. Your doctor might add a nasal spray if antihistamines **don't** work alone. This spray might have a corticosteroid. (See "Controller Medicine – Inhaled Corticosteroids," page 57.)

What should I keep in mind?

- Young children can have allergy symptoms all year long from allergens in the home.
- Older children get hay fever from spring and fall pollens.
- A nasal allergy might cause ear and sinus infections. (See "Sinus Infection," page 122.)
- A nasal allergy can make asthma harder to control.

What can I do at home?

- Remove asthma triggers from your home.
- Give your child the medicine the doctor has told you to give.

- Do what the doctor has told you to do for your child.
- Tell your whole family how to care for your child.

When do I call the doctor or nurse?

- Call if you think your child has hay fever.
- Call if you need medicine to give your child.
- Call when you **don't** know what to do for your child.
- Call if your child **doesn't** get better with medicine.

Sinus Infection

What is it?

When a child's sinuses are inflamed or infected, the sinuses **don't** drain.

What should I know?

Sinuses are air pockets in the bones of the face and head. The sinuses open into the nose. Another name for sinus infection is "sinusitis."

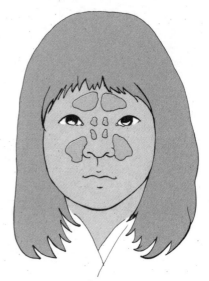

Problems in a child's sinuses will make asthma worse. Your child might **not** say they have pain. But they might have some of these signs:

- Stuffy nose
- Yellow or green mucus from the nose
- Fever
- Swelling around the eyes
- Coughing at night
- Acting cranky
- Headache in an older child

Sinus Infection

Sinus infection usually comes 10-14 days after a cold. The signs of infection might last many weeks. They make your child's asthma worse.

Take your child to a doctor. Your doctor might:

- X-ray the sinuses.
- Tell you what to do for your child.
- Have your child take an antibiotic (ann-tie-bye-**ot**-ic) for up to 3 weeks.

What should I keep in mind?

- Sinus problems can make asthma worse.
- A sinus infection can become chronic and last for months.
- A nasal allergy can lead to a chronic sinus infection.
- Take your child to the doctor.

What can I do at home?

- Use a salt water nasal spray to clear mucus from the nose. You can buy the spray at the drug store. The doctor might tell you to use a medicine dropper with salt water instead.

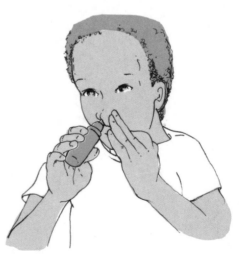

- Give your child the medicine the doctor has told you to give.

- Do what the doctor has told you to do for your child.
- Tell your family how to care for your child.
- Give **all** the antibiotic to your child. **Don't** stop when your child seems better.

When do I call the doctor or nurse?

- Call if you think your child has a sinus infection.
- Call if you need medicine to give your child.
- Call when you **don't** know what to do for your child.
- Call if your child **doesn't** get better with medicine.

Living with Asthma 7

Notes

Doctor Visits

What is it?

Get the most from visits with your child's doctor.

What should I know?

Keep doctor appointments even when your child seems healthy. Bring with you:

- Your child's inhalers.
- Your child's Asthma Action Plan.
- Questions you want to ask the doctor. (See below for ideas.)

Be ready to answer these questions:

- How many times a week:
  - Has your child had asthma signs during the day?
  - Has your child had asthma signs in the night?
  - How often does your child use quick-relief medicine (**not** counting pre-treatment for exercise)?
- How many days of school or day care has your child missed?
- How often does your child take controller medicine?
- Does your child have asthma signs when playing or doing exercise?
- Has your child been:
  - To the emergency room since their last doctor visit?

- Admitted to the hospital (kept overnight) for asthma since their last visit?

- What things or places seem to make your child's asthma worse?

- What have your child's peak flow meter numbers been since the last visit?

- Do you think your child's asthma is better or worse since the last visit?

Write down questions for the doctor **before** your visit. Bring them with you. You might want to ask:

- Why has my child's asthma changed since last time?

- What does my child need to do at school?

- Are there any changes in the Asthma Action Plan?

- What could be making my child's asthma worse?

- Are we using the inhalers the right way?

- What should I do in an emergency?

- When should I bring my child in again?

Make sure you have enough refills to last until your next visit.

What should I keep in mind?

- It's important to work with your doctor to control your child's asthma.

- Your time with the doctor might be short.

- The best thing you can do is be ready for the visit.

- Be ready to tell the doctor about your child's asthma. This helps the doctor know what to do for your child.

It's a good idea to have a well-child asthma check-up every year.

What can I do at home?

- If you can, plan for **all** guardians to go with your child to the doctor.
- Talk to your child about the doctor visit. Tell your child what the doctor will do.
- Ask your child if they have any questions for the doctor.
- Have your child help get ready for the doctor visit.
- Pack up these things to take to the doctor visit:
  - Asthma Action Plan
  - All asthma medicines and inhalers
  - Mask or holding chamber
  - Best peak flow numbers
  - List of your questions

When do I call the doctor or nurse?

- Call when you need an appointment.
- Call if you **can't** keep an appointment.
- Call anytime you have a question.
- Call when you **don't** understand how to care for your child.
- Call if you **can't** do what the doctor told you to do.

Asthma at Day Care

What is it?

Other people care for your child at day care. Be sure they **all** know what to do for your child's asthma.

What should I know?

Everyone who works at your child's day care needs to know about your child's asthma. This includes office staff, caregivers, and anyone who spends time with your child.

Before your child goes to day care:

- Go see the staff and caregivers to talk to them about your child.

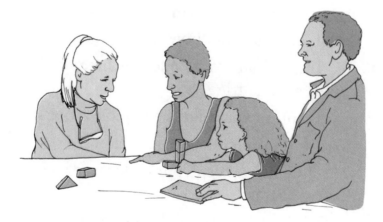

- Ask your child's day care for a form your doctor can sign. This form says it's OK to give your child quick-relief medicine.

- Give the day care a copy of your child's Asthma Action Plan.

Things to ask at day care:

- Who will be giving medicine to my child?
- Where will you keep the medicine? (Your child might need medicine right away.)

Things to give day care staff:

- Your child's Asthma Action Plan
- Phone numbers for calling you
- Names and phone numbers to call when your child's asthma gets worse
- A quick-relief inhaler for your child
- A holding chamber, and a mask if your child uses them
- A peak flow meter if your child is older than age 5

Things to tell people working at day care:

- Teach day care staff how to give medicine to your child.
- Tell them about your child's asthma. Tell them your child's asthma triggers.
- Tell them if your child is allergic to foods or animals.
- Talk about exercise for your child.
    - Tell them to keep your child inside when it's smoggy, very hot, or very cold.
    - Tell them if your child uses an inhaler 5-15 minutes before exercise.
- **For a bad attack, tell them to call 911 and then call you.**

What should I keep in mind?

- You need to help the day care prepare to take care of your child. They need to know what to do when your child has asthma signs.

- Make sure they have the Asthma Action Plan. Make sure they understand how to use it.

- Your child's asthma can be controlled at day care. Your child will be able to do what the other children do.

- Check with the day care often to see how your child is doing.

- Talk to teachers to make sure your child **isn't** being left out. Find ways for your child to join in activities. If your child **can't** play a game, they can keep score.

What can I do at home?

- Mark everything that goes to day care with your child's name, medicine name, and how often to use it.

- You need to keep track of doses in the inhaler at day care. Give them a new inhaler when you think they need one.

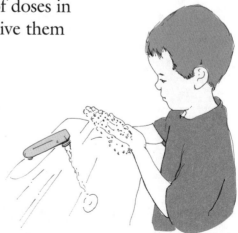

- Teach your child **not** to share inhalers with other children.

- Teach your child to wash their hands often.

- Keep your child home from day care when:

- Your child has had a restless night with coughing or wheezing.
- Your child is breathing faster than normal.
- Your child **doesn't** seem well.

When do I call the doctor or nurse?

- Call to ask if your child should go to day care.
- Call if you **don't** have an Asthma Action Plan to give your child's day care.
- Call if your child is having trouble with asthma at day care.

Asthma at School

What is it?

Your child might have asthma signs at school. Other people care for your child at school. Be sure the school staff knows what to do for your child's asthma.

What should I know?

Everyone who works at the school needs to know about your child's asthma. Tell these people:

- Principal
- School nurse
- Teachers and substitute teachers
- PE coach (gym teacher)
- Counselors
- Bus driver
- Anyone who spends time with your child

Before your child goes to school:

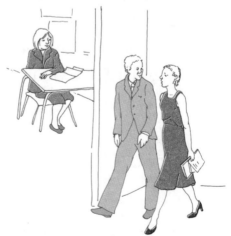

- Go to see the teachers, nurses, and staff at the school. Talk to them about your child. Do this at the start of each school year.
- Ask the school for a form your doctor can sign.

133

This form says it's OK to give your child quick-relief medicine.

- Give the school a copy of your child's Asthma Action Plan.

Things to ask at school:

- Who will be giving medicine to my child?
- Do they know how to give the medicine?
- Where will you keep the medicine? (Your child might need medicine right away.)

Things to give school staff:

- Your child's Asthma Action Plan
- Phone numbers for calling you
- Names and phone numbers to call when your child's asthma gets worse
- A quick-relief inhaler for your child
- A holding chamber and mask if your child uses them

Things to tell the people working at school:

- Tell them about your child's asthma. Tell them your child's asthma triggers.
- Tell them if your child is allergic to foods or animals.
- Talk about exercise for your child.
  - Tell them to keep your child inside when it's smoggy, very hot, or very cold.
  - Tell them if your child uses an inhaler 5-15 minutes before exercise.
- **For a bad attack, tell them to call 911 and then call you.**

What should I keep in mind?

- Your school will give you a form for you and the doctor to sign. This form says it's OK for the school to give your child quick-relief medicine.

- You also need to give the school your child's Asthma Action Plan.

- You need to help the school prepare to take care of your child. They need to know what to do when your child has asthma signs.

- Make sure they have the Asthma Action Plan. Make sure they understand how to use it.

- Your child's asthma can be controlled at school. Your child will be able to do what the other children do.

- Talk to teachers to make sure your child **isn't** being left out. Find a way for your child to be a part of activities. If your child **can't** play a game, have your child keep score.

- Make sure your child is **not** being teased at school because of their asthma. Have the teacher talk to the class about asthma.

What can I do at home?

- Put your child's name on their inhaler, and anything else for school. Keep a copy of your child's Asthma Action Plan with the medicine. The plan will tell how to give the medicine.

- Keep track of doses in the inhaler that's at school. Tell the school to let you know each time your child uses the inhaler. Give them a new inhaler when you think they need one.

- Check with the school often to see how your child is doing.

- When you sign a permission slip for your child to go on a field trip, send back a note with it. Mention your child's asthma in the note. Make sure the school and all teachers know how to reach you or your child's doctor. This is extra important if the field trip is to a zoo or farm.

- Teach your child **not** to share inhalers with other children.

- Teach your child to wash their hands often at school.

- **Don't** send your child to school when:
  - Quick-relief medicine **didn't** relieve asthma signs.
  - Your child is having trouble breathing.
  - You're worried about how well your child is breathing.
  - Your child had a restless night with coughing or wheezing.

When do I call the doctor or nurse?

- Call if you're **not** sure if your child should stay home from school.
- Call when you need a signed copy of your child's Asthma Action Plan for school.
- Call when you need the doctor to sign any forms. For example, you'll need a paper saying it's OK for the school to give your child medicine.
- Call if your child is having trouble with asthma at school.

Word List

A

- **acid reflux**—When food in the stomach comes back up the throat.

- **airways**—Tubes that bring air into and out of the lungs.

- **albuterol**—A quick-relief medicine that relieves asthma right away. Generic name for medicine commonly used for asthma.

- **allergen**—Anything that can cause an allergy. Allergens in the air might cause asthma signs.

- **Asthma Action Plan**—A plan the doctor writes for you and your child. The plan tells what to do every day and when your child's asthma gets worse. Your child's signs of asthma and peak flow meter number are used to tell what medicine to give.

- **asthma attack**—When the signs of asthma happen all at once. Sometimes called a flare-up or an episode.

- **asthma control**—When your child can play, sleep, go to school, and do what other children do. Peak flow numbers are normal. Quick-relief medicine is almost never needed.

- **asthma signs**—Things you can feel, see, or hear in your child that tell you about their asthma. Also called "symptoms."

B

- **BM (bowel movement)**—Solid waste passed out of the body.

- **bronchial asthma**—Medical name for asthma.

- **bronchial tubes**—Large tubes for air to move in and out of the lungs.

- **bronchodilators**—Medicines that open the airways. Also called quick-relief medicines.

C

- **chronic**—Happens all the time. Might get better, but never goes away.

- **Color Zone System**—Uses traffic light colors to tell you what to do for your child.

- **controller medicine—Doesn't** give relief right away. Taken daily to prevent the signs of asthma. Reduces redness and swelling in the airways and lungs.

D

- **dust mite**—A kind of very tiny bug. It lives in dust all over a house. Lives in bedrooms, pillows, carpets, drapes, and mattresses. Causes allergies and asthma signs in children.

- **dry powder inhaler**—Small tool that has a dry powder medicine in it. Your child breathes the medicine into their lungs.

Word List

E

- **Exercise-induced asthma**—A diagnosis a doctor makes when a child has asthma during or after exercise. Also called EIA.

G

- **Green Color Zone**—No signs of asthma. Asthma is well controlled.

H

- **holding chamber**—A long tube connected to an inhaler. It holds the sprayed medicine while the child breathes it in.

I

- **important**—Give it your full attention.
- **inflammation**—When the airways get red and swollen. Causes coughing, wheezing, and trouble breathing.
- **inhaler**—A small tool used to put medicine in the lungs when you breathe in. A "dry powder inhaler" sprays a fine powder. A "metered-dose inhaler" sprays a mist.
- **intermittent**—When your child has asthma only once in awhile.
- **irritants**—Things in the air that can cause an asthma attack. These include cigarette smoke, cold air, smog, and strong smells.

M

- **mask**—Worn over the mouth and nose to help a young child breathe in the full dose of medicine.

- **MDI**—Metered-dose inhaler. A tool with medicine in it. The MDI uses a gas to make mist, which the child breathes in.

- **mold**—Grows in damp and wet places. Easy to breathe in. Often triggers asthma.

- **mucus**—A thick liquid the body makes. Mucus protects the nose, mouth, throat, airways, and lungs. Allergens and infections can bring on too much mucus. Too much mucus will block the airways.

N

- **nebulizer**—A machine that changes liquid medicine to a mist that your child breathes in.

P

- **peak flow meter**—Used by most children 5 years old and older. Can help you tell if your child's asthma symptoms are getting worse.

- **personal best peak flow number**—Highest peak flow meter number when a child **doesn't** have signs of asthma.

- **pollen**—An allergen shed by flowers and plants in the spring and fall.

Q

- **quick-relief medicines**—Asthma medicines like albuterol that work right away when a child has coughing, wheezing, or trouble breathing.

Word List

R

- **Red Color Zone**—Asthma signs and peak flow number are in the danger zone. Emergency help is needed right away.

S

- **severe**—The worst.
- **side effect**—When a medicine does something to the body other than what the medicine is for.
- **spirometry**—Used in a doctor's office or a clinic to measure how well a child is breathing. It might be used to diagnose asthma.
- **swollen**—Puffy.
- **symptom**—Something that you feel, see, or hear from a child that **isn't** normal. The symptom tells you something's wrong.

T

- **trigger**—Anything that can cause a child to have signs of asthma.

W

- **wheezing or whistling sound**—Usually heard when a child breathes out. This means the airways are blocked.

Y

- **Yellow Color Zone**—Watch for signs of asthma getting worse. Give quick-relief medicine. Your child might be taking a controller medicine every day.

Z

- **zone**—Matched to the colors of the traffic light (green, yellow, and red). Used to tell you which asthma medicine to use and what to do.

What's in This Book from A to Z

145

What's in This Book from A to Z

People We Want to Thank

We wish to thank the following people for their help with this book:

Albert E. Barnett, M.D.

William Berger, M.D.

Cristina Bernal

Gina Capaldi

Blanca M. Castro

Maria Collis

Sherwin Gillman, M.D.

Alan B. Goldsobel, M.D.

Warren Hand

Gabriela Hernandez

Yoly Herrera

Rose Loaiza

Vanessa E. Loera

Donna McKenzie, CFNP

Olga Molina

Marla Nathan

Ruby Raya-Morones, M.D.

Audrey Riffenburgh

Vanessa Rodriguez

Nancy Rushton, R.N.

Marian Ryan, Ph.D., MPH, CHES

Arely Servin

Michael Villaire

Carolyn Wendt

Other Books in the Series

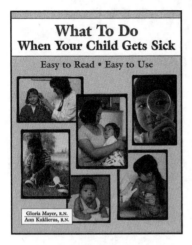

ISBN 978-0-9701245-0-0
$12.95

What To Do When Your Child Gets Sick*

There are many things you can do at home for your child. At last, an easy to read, easy to use book written by 2 nurses. This book tells you:

- What to look for when your child is sick.
- When to call the doctor.
- How to take your child's temperature.
- What to do when your child has the flu.
- How to care for cuts and scrapes.
- What to feed your child when he or she is sick.
- How to stop the spread of infection.
- How to prevent accidents around your home.
- What to do in an emergency.

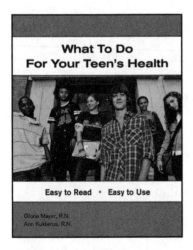

ISBN 978-0-9720148-9-2
$12.95

What To Do For Your Teen's Health

The teen years are hard on parents and teens. There are many things you can do to help your teen. At last, an easy to read, easy to use book written by 2 nurses. This book tells you:

- About the body changes that happen to teens.
- How to get ready for the teen years.
- How to talk with your teen.
- What you can do to feel closer to your teen.
- How to help your teen do well in school.
- All about dating and sex.
- How to keep your teen safe.
- The signs of trouble and where to go for help.

Also available in Spanish.
*Also available in Vietnamese, Chinese, and Korean.
To order, call (800) 434-4633 or visit www.iha4health.org.

Other Books in the Series

What To Do
When You're Having a Baby

There are many things a woman can do to have a healthy baby. Here's an easy to read, easy to use book written by 2 nurses that tells you:

- How to get ready for pregnancy.
- About the health care you need during pregnancy.
- Things you should not do when you are pregnant.
- How to take care of yourself so you have a healthy baby.
- Body changes you will have each month.
- Simple things you can do to feel better.
- Warning signs of problems and what to do about them.
- All about labor and delivery.
- How to feed and care for your new baby.

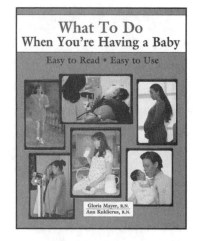

ISBN 978-0-9835976-0-5
$12.95

What To Do
For Senior Health*

There are many things that you can do to take charge of your health during your senior years. This book tells about:

- Body changes that come with aging.
- Common health problems of seniors.
- Things to consider about health insurance.
- How to choose a doctor and where to get health care.
- Buying and taking medicines.
- Simple things you can do to prevent falls and accidents.
- What you can do to stay healthy.

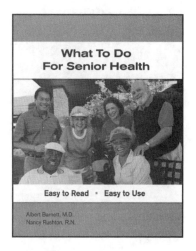

ISBN 978-0-9701245-4-8
$12.95

Also available in Spanish.
*Also available in Vietnamese.
To order, call (800) 434-4633 or visit www.iha4health.org.

Other Books in the Series

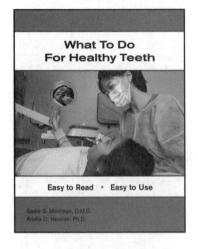

ISBN 978-0-9721048-0-9
$12.95

What To Do
For Healthy Teeth

It is important to take good care of your teeth from an early age. This book tells how to do that. It also explains all about teeth, gums, and how dentists work with you to keep your teeth healthy, including:

- How to care for your teeth and gums.
- What you need to care for your teeth and gums.
- Caring for your teeth when you're having a baby.
- Caring for your child's teeth.
- When to call the dentist.
- What to expect at a dental visit.
- Dental care needs for seniors.
- What to do if you hurt your mouth or teeth.

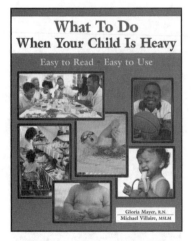

ISBN 978-0-9721048-4-7
$12.95

What To Do
When Your Child Is Heavy

There are many things you can do to help your heavy child live a healthy lifestyle. Here's an easy to read, easy to use book that tells you:

- How to tell if your child is heavy.
- How to shop and pay for healthy food.
- Dealing with your heavy child's feelings and self-esteem.
- How to read the Nutrition Facts Label.
- Healthy breakfasts, lunches, and dinners.
- Correct portion sizes.
- Why exercise is so important.
- Tips for eating healthy when you eat out.
- Information on diabetes and other health problems of heavy children.

Also available in Spanish.
To order, call (800) 434-4633or visit www.iha4health.org.